DON'T CUT MY LIFE-LINE

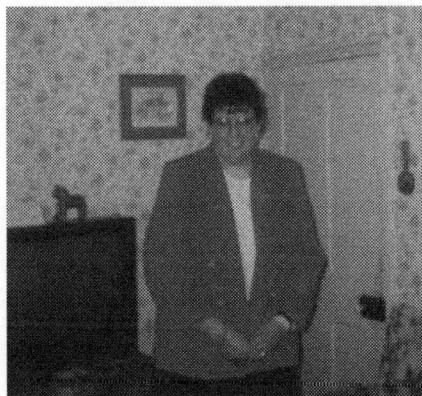

JO

RAINBOW

'One million people commit suicide every year'
The World Heath Organization

Published by:
Chipmunkapublishing
PO Box 6872
Brentwood
Essex
CM13 1ZT
United Kingdom

http://www.chipmunkapublishing.com

Copyright © 2007 Jo Rainbow

Additional material by Gary A. Ayres and Chris Farmer
Proof-read by Becky Barrett

ISBN 9781847471109

This book is dedicated to...

My psychiatrist, Dr. Smith, for his patience in building trust. For believing I have a future.

For all members, past and present of the evening group, for helping me understand that the tangled mass of blackness inside is feelings. For listening, accepting and showing me love. Most of all thank you for staying. For years I thought the pain I felt inside was destructive. That the only way I could survive was to lash out in anger...mostly at myself. Thank you for showing me love, compassion and hope for a new life...built on love.

Tony, art therapist... whose wisdom and understanding inspired this book.

All the doctors and staff, who took the time to see a person behind the battered, screwed up person I used to be.

For my family and friends, thank you for staying with me. For loving me and holding on and for endless mugs of tea.

For Pete, 'To dream good dreams think of flying.' Pete helped me break the terrible secrecy that surrounds self-injury. Thank you for listening, accepting me with unconditional love.

Most of all, this book is for you. May you find the courage and love needed to heal your pain. With love from one who has survived years of self-injury and is learning to live.

With all my heart I send you love, Jo Rainbow, author 2003.

CHAPTER ONE

Identifying The Problem

My heart pounds as I leap up the stairs, three at a time. My thoughts are racing. I have to get there before they hurt her.

'Gran. It's Jo.' I lower the cot sides. Gran smiles, yet her usually bright eyes are watery. I stroke Gran's fluffy white hair; she leans towards me.

'Jo...'

'I love you Gran. I've come to take you home.'

'Mrs Evans, your medication.'

I fold my legs around the chair as a nurse pushes her trolley next to Gran's bed. I feel my body tense, rage boils inside, yet before I can find words, the nurse is gone. I pull the thin curtains round to keep out nosey nurses. Gran has lived for ninety years without the need for hospitals. As for tablets, a drop of brandy in her tea is Gran's remedy. The noise is constant: clattering, whirring machines, people chattering, laughing around the next bed. I rest my head next to Gran's and catch the faint, familiar smell of lavender as she closes her eyes.

'I'll get you home tomorrow Gran.'

'We don't need these closed.'

A rotund lady sweeps the curtains back.

'Nice cup of tea dear.'

'No, that can't be for my Gran.'

I stand and glare at the tea lady. She brushes past me and wraps Gran's hands around the plastic feeding cup.

'Drink your tea sweetheart.'

'My Gran has hot tea, in a china teacup with two shortbread biscuits.'

The woman snorted.

'Mrs Evans must drink plenty of fluids.' she said as she left.

Gran's hands shake; she spills some of the liquid on my hand.

'That's not tea. It's horrible, lukewarm dregs.' Gran nods and hands me the cup.

'Aunt Betty had tea with us today. It wasn't the same without you.'

'Missed my sponge cake?' Gran chuckles, her eyes sparkle then fade.

'Come home with me Gran. I could get a wheelchair…'

Nurses' chatter breaks my thoughts.

'Shame about old Mrs Evans.'

'Collapsed at home?'

'Cancer…'

'Excuse me' I call out.

One of the nurses turns. I stare back at her as she takes in my torn jeans and paint-smudged t-shirt.

'Can I help?'

'I need to know… to know if Gran… '

'Yes?'

'Another pillow?'

I hate myself as I sit back down. Why couldn't I ask for help? I look at Gran. She seems so tiny and vulnerable in her white hospital gown.

I remember lying in hospital. My young body was shaking in fear as I lost my dignity to a barrage of tests. The doctor told me to be brave. I didn't cry. I had no more tears to cry. I have to save Gran from that. I wrap my arms around Gran and rest my head on her shoulders. Tears burn my eyes. I don't cry. I learned not to cry a long time ago. We hold each other in silence in this sterile environment. The latest technology bleeps, buzzes, announcing its intention to save lives, yet Gran is fading fast. I stand, look from Gran to the door.

'What can I do?'

The next day, I run home from college, mother is standing on the doorstep. She fingers her silver crucifix, eyes downcast. Her lips move in silent prayer and I know something terrible has happened.

'Jo… Gran died.'

I push past my mother, slam the kettle on to boil. It whistles as neighbours crowd in.

'Such a shock.'

'Blessing, lovely way to go, she died in her sleep?'

<u>Saying goodbye</u>

A funeral service is a traditional part of our grieving for loved ones. It may also be appropriate to say goodbye in other ways too. Perhaps by visiting a place where you have happy memories of your loved one, by writing a letter to say those things you wish you could have said or by holding onto treasured memories of your loved one with photographs, trinkets and ornaments.

We can also suffer grief at the break up of a relationship or marriage, or job loss.

The small village church is packed for Gran's funeral. My family stand at the front. Father is wearing his best suit. Mother clasps lace-gloved hands together. Her sister Betty stands tall, her hands trembling as she clutches the service sheet. I never wear dresses but today I have a new black dress. I stare at the pine coffin.
'The Lord's My Shepherd, I'll not want, He makes me down to lie.' I'm suddenly aware everyone else is singing...
'In pastures green he leadeth me, the quiet waters by.'
I stare in silence at the wreath on the pine coffin. Mother dabs at her eyes with a lace handkerchief. Father blows his nose vigorously. I wish I could cry. Gran's funeral is followed by more pots of tea and I wonder if it is possible to drown grief.

<u>The pain of silence</u>

After the loss of a loved one it's natural to cry, talk, shout and even scream. Grief is easier to live through if we can share and express our feelings but I'm already used to keeping quiet. For years I've buried my feelings. I don't think I even have feelings anymore. I've pushed feelings away since I was a young child and it has become an automatic reflex now. Whenever I start to feel, I shut out the sensations and block what my body is trying to communicate.
During this time I carry on as usual... grief and loss is nothing new to me. Our family has had six deaths over the last

two years, yet Gran held us together. Every day I walk to Gran's. Halfway through her garden gate I scream inside, the empty house screams back and echoes with the pain I feel. Years of pent up emotion build into an internal volcano. One day it may erupt. One day the feelings will burst out, destroying others and myself. This is why I have to keep my feelings locked in. I'm scared to let out even a little of what I feel in case I contaminate others with my evil; the evil mass that my blocked feelings have turned into. I now understand that feelings are comfortable or uncomfortable, they are not bad or evil.

Grief is not a tidy process; we all go through the stages of shock, denial, anger, guilt, relief, sadness, despair and anxiety. Eventually readjustment is possible, built on acceptance and strength from cherished memories.

My search begins to fill the void left the day Gran died. Grief and loss is nothing new to me, yet Gran had always held my family together. Gran was my refuge, my best friend, and my reason for living.

<u>Difficult choices</u>

Many people can identify with feeling lost, especially after the death of a loved one. We have a choice. To face reality or to run and hide from our feelings. The grieving process can be seen as stages of questions and feelings. Initial denial. Why me? Why did they have to die? Anger, sadness, acceptance. Finally moving on, taking our loved ones' cherished memories with us. We cope in the best way we can at the time. There is no right or wrong way but it helps to allow yourself time to grieve.

A college trip is planned for the winter half-term. The bright lights and constant noise of London is an exciting distraction from the desperate silence that has filled my home since Gran died. Painfully shy, I keep to the edge of the group of students, trailing round museums and galleries. The last night of our stay two students organise a party. A group of Russian students had arrived earlier that day. Excitement is tangible as the music system is rigged up and balloons and streamers pinned up. Students anxiously change.

'This all right?'

'Oh Jo, at least put on make-up.'

'Vodka?'

I look up into a stranger's deep blue eyes. A moment's hesitation and I down the fiery liquid in one.

'Good? My name Stavos, name you?'

Stavos squeezes in next to me. I smile at his crop of unruly black hair, meet his dark eyes. With ease he slips his arm round my shoulder. The stranger's warmth mixed with the vodka melts any inhibitions I may have had.

Later that evening, the basement room vibrates as music blares. On the edge of the room I notice the teacher watching Stavos and me dancing a little closer than is proper, or is that the dim lights? No need to worry about Jo anyway.

Touch says more than words...

'I know English little,' he said.

I hug Stavos closer, could this be love?

'Come.'

Stavos leads me up the winding staircase to his room. Huddled together on his bed, he shows me pictures of his hometown. I rest my head on his chest and breathe in his musk aftershave.

'Friends?'

I kiss Stavos lightly on his forehead. He grabs me roughly. His hands form a grip of cold steel. His breath hot, panting. Blinded by tears of frustration and fear I slam the door behind me. Outside in the cool night air, I feel a warmth brush my hair.

'Sorry'

Stavos and I walk through London streets, neon lights flash adverts, strange purple smoke billows out from all night cafes. We hold hands, marvelling at this city which never sleeps. Dawn breaks. Smells of freshly baked bread awaken hunger in us.

Stavos presses his hand to the train window as if to wipe away my tears. To jeers and taunts of fellow students I wave goodbye. Hold me, hold me, the train rattles to a steady rhythm of pain and loss.

I hold memories of Stavos close. If I'd been prettier, if I'd given him what he wanted would he have stayed?

Broken hearted

Grief and loss takes time to heal. We all need time to go through the natural stages of grieving. Death is a part of our lives, yet it's natural to feel sad, to cry. At this time I'm still mourning the loss of my Gran. Gran was my life. Every day I'd spend time with Gran, baking, sewing, chatting over cups of tea. Gran's death left emptiness in my life. I began searching for love to fill this void on my trip to London.

Gran loved and accepted everyone who came to her door with an open heart and fresh baked biscuits. After my experience with Stavos I questioned whether love is freely given in an adult world. I started to question myself. Did I deserve love? Was I acceptable? Through this time I'm also becoming aware of a gnawing pain inside. I feel isolated, alone. I feel lonely without Gran.
I'm reaching out in desperation for someone to fill the void. My feelings are so intense I feel trapped.

My village home seems quiet, claustrophobic. I'm longing for escape. I leap at an unexpected opportunity to join a hiking expedition to the Lake District. The college party is one short. Walking is one exercise I enjoy, no embarrassment at having to change in communal changing rooms. There's also the added excitement of the confident young man joining our party from the next village.
'He's so... so nice.'
'Get real Jo. You haven't got a chance with Paul.'
'I wasn't thinking of...'
'Get on with packing Jo, or we'll miss the train.'

Scrambling up the shingle, sharp rocks pierce blistered feet. I stretch, hold onto Paul's hand. Through the increasing mist the peak of Helvellyn taunts weary climbers.
'Nearly there.'

Paul's confidence inspires me. Finally at the Mountain peak, sheltering from biting winds in a stone shelter, I squeeze in next to Paul. Icy fingers tear at chunks of bread and cheese.

'Come on, time to move' the leader shouts.

'Let's go Paul. Going down is easy.'

I confidently stride out, determined to impress my new friend. The only pathway forms a ridge that cuts swirling grey mist like a razor. I freeze in fear, bumped forward by eager hikers. I stumble and fall, falling into blackness. Sharp stones tear my trousers, releasing warm blood, sticky to touch.

'Jo, be brave,' Paul shouts.

I pull myself back up, thoughts racing.

Later that evening Paul strokes my head as we sit squeezed in a stairway corner.

'Did well today, locals are saying the weather is the worst they've seen for months.'

I lean my aching body against Paul, feel his strong arms holding me.

'I thought you'd cry when you fell. You're brave Jo.'

Paul looks away. I feel his body tremor.

'You okay?'

'Thinking about my Grandad. He died two weeks ago.'

'My Gran died recently too.'

I hug Paul, too choked to say more. Minutes pass as I relax in his arms.

During the train journey home, I admire Paul's muscular build and mane of golden hair. He will be the perfect father to my eight children. I've chosen names already... Elizabeth, Roger, Thomas. One thing at a time. What to buy Paul for Christmas?

Christmas isn't as I planned. It's three o'clock by the time we find time to be alone. I cry. I cry for Gran, for my fear of rejection. In desperation I cling to Paul. He is my refuge, my best friend and by the time we find a bed-sit, my lover.

Every day I hurry home from work to be with Paul, we play his Beatles records, I talk about Gran...

One evening Paul snaps at me.

'Let go Jo. Your Gran's dead. It's time to move on.'
'It's not only losing Gran…'
'What's troubling you Jo?'
Paul's voice softens.
'Nothing' I said, pushing him away.

<u>When there are no words…</u>

It's important to feel ready to talk, for you to take control.
Trust builds slowly, especially when you have been let down or
felt betrayed. Try building trust slowly. Try sharing how you feel
first if events are too painful or personal to talk about at the start.
If you can't find words because you can't identify feelings, start
becoming aware of your body. Headaches, stomach pain may
indicate tension or repressed anger. General aches and
tiredness, depression or sadness. Learn to listen to your body. It
is giving you messages as feelings throughout the day. You
could also try writing, drawing or painting what you feel. If you
like, you could share this with a trusted friend or nurse.

Maybe I could talk to Paul?

The nightmares return that night. Mocking voices scream.
'Bad girl, you made mummy ill. You're to blame.'
I know I must keep my past secret. If Paul found out, he would
leave.

In the months that follow, I try hard to move on. I throw myself
into work, decorating our bed-sit and making wedding plans.

One blustery March morning, my best friend Susan and me
are wedding dress hunting.
'Help! I look huge!'
I emerge from the fitting rooms like a reject from ballet school,
covered in waves of pink froth.
'Something simple?'
I settle for a plain white, traditional dress.
'You'll still phone when you're away?' I ask.
'Yeah sure, it's only Scotland, not the end of the world.'

'For three years!'

'I'll be home for the holidays.'

I hug Susan as we part. Deep inside I sense that Susan is starting a new life, one that I'm no longer part of.

Three weeks left to our wedding, I can't understand the pain I feel inside. Clean, have to keep busy. I race around with the Hoover tearing at the threadbare carpets. Table and chairs gleam under a thick layer of polish. I juggle pots and pans and chop vegetables.

'I must have a meal ready for Paul'

Paul isn't due home yet. Paul. I tremble, curl into his armchair. My body shakes with pain. I can't marry Paul. I love Susan. I'm bad, evil. Bad girls cry. Bad children go to hell. Inside my head voices scream, memories pierce blackness. I know one last desperate escape route, last used when Gran died. I break three glasses, scattering splinters over the sink. Self-injury is my dark, secret tool of survival.

The legacy of secrets

I remember that summer's day, the first time I self-injured. Words flashed hotter than the midday sun. Doors slammed, pots and pans crashed across the kitchen. I wish my parents would stop shouting at each other. From my room window I watch Gran's house, see Gran drawing the bedroom curtains for her afternoon nap. Voices rage downstairs, I pick up my sewing, the lace runner I'm making for Gran. I trim loose threads, trace the scissors over my hand. Gran's scissors, my hands. As if watching a film I see myself draw blood. The tiny beads of blood match the lace pattern. I am in control. This is my body.

Basic first aid

It is important to check wounds, especially if you have been dissociated, that is unaware of events during the act of injury. Ensure the wound is cleaned, kept clean and dry. If the wound is gaping or blistered, seek medical attention. If this is difficult, take a friend for support. Following an act of injury you may feel shocked, distressed, numb, high, any number of different feelings. Take time to consider your emotional needs. For example, have a cup of tea, play music, write how you feel, take a nap.

My cutting expresses my deepest hurt. No words, no tears yet my wound cries. From deep within a silent scream emerges, I find release, peace. I have taken control of my body. Tending my wound gives me comfort.

Hours later Paul flings open the door.

'Jo. Jo what happened?'

I stagger to my feet. Blood drips, silent, silent as the screaming in my head.

'Bad day at work'

I can't explain. I feel trapped. If Paul found out, he wouldn't love me. I'd be alone. Abandoned.

I feel safe with Paul. Love at any cost? When Paul holds me, when he tells me, 'I'll take care of you,' I know he loves me. Inside, I still doubt him, does he really love me?

How can you love me? I don't even know who I am!

My doubts about Paul's love for me echo in my head long after my arm has healed. How can he possibly love me? I've always been bad. I was so bad mummy got ill. I was never good enough to make mummy better. She was still sad when I left home, now I've hurt her again. Caring for a loved one is rewarding, also exhausting. Imagine you are five years old, holding mummy's hand, wiping her tears away. Listening to words that have no meaning. Mummy keeps crying. Big tears splash on my pink dungarees. I cry too. I want to make mummy happy. Years of caring, sharing, bonding so close. I'm no longer a person.

The first time I self-injured I found a way to survive. This time I'd found a way of drawing boundaries. Marking my body claimed it back for me. I still didn't know who I was, but the mass evil inside at least had a defining wall, my skin.

Making a fresh start...

If you are an active self-injurer and are trying to stop, start with basics. Is your environment safe? Is your home, or room, a friendly and safe place to be? Could you decorate your room to your own tastes? Posters, teddy bears, rugs, cushions, candles are just some ideas to add enjoyment to your living areas. It is also important to take care of your physical needs, eat five fruit or vegetables per day. Exercise, even a twenty minute walk is beneficial. Be positive. Tell yourself you are wonderful. Really, you are!

Look in the mirror and see a princess

- You are unique
- You are special
- You are a brave and strong person
- You are a kind and loving person
- You are intelligent
- Every day you make progress

Summary.

Feelings can only be locked away for so long. Some form of expression is needed for survival. When Gran died I couldn't name my feelings. If it is difficult to identify your feelings, start by listening to your body. Physical pain, nightmares and flashbacks are often the body's way of expressing pent up feelings.

If you are an active self-injurer, please remember your safety first. If in any doubt seek medical advice for wounds. This is vital if you have been dissociated, that is, unaware of events. You may have caused more damage than intended.

Crisis tips:
- When feelings start to build to a point where you feel uncomfortable, phone the Samaritans, or draw, paint or write what you feel. If you injure yourself later, this may still lessen the damage done.

- Remember you are worth fighting for. You are a unique, special person. When I started to self-injure, as destructive as it sounds I was still fighting to survive. If you're afraid to even think about stopping self-injury, please keep reading. This book is about making choices, not forcing you into decisions.

Crisis coping tips:

- First aid: Remember to clean wounds carefully. If necessary seek medical attention.
- Phone the Samaritans.
- Instead of self-harming, treat yourself.
- Play music.

CHAPTER TWO

Silent Screams Echo in Dark Nights

The first months of our marriage are the fairytale I've dreamed of. I have a new job, Paul is promoted to supervisor at his office. His longer hours mean my plans to start a family are put on hold but I continue to decorate our bed-sit, making a nest for the children to come.

'This is my best summer ever.'

I gaze up at Paul, soaking up the last rays of sun.

'Tell me another story.'

'In a magical time there was a beautiful princess. One day...'

I lay my head on Paul's lap. Sun burns pink, fades into a golden sky.

'Come on Jo.'

Paul shakes me awake.

'It's my work's charity ball tonight.'

'It's Annie's engagement dance too.'

'Annie?'

'Orange hair'

I mumble, struggling into my jeans.

'My supervisor at work.'

'I remember now. I've seen her at the shops, nice girl, always friendly.'

'She's my best friend.' I announce proudly.

My only friend, I add silently to myself.

'At least it gives me an excuse to leave the office do early.'

The evening passes slowly, endless speeches, toasts and coffee follow the meal. Much as I admire Paul's commitment to his firm, I'm grateful to leave the stuffed suits behind. We run for the last taxi, laughing as Paul flings his tie out of the window.

Disco lights flash, the crowded dance floor vibrates to music and tapping feet. I'm idling at the end of the bar, waiting for Paul to return with our drinks.

'Hi Jo. You look as keen as me. I don't like playing sardines to Rap music either.'

'Hi. Sam isn't it?'

I look up at the stranger. Black curly hair, dark twinkling eyes laugh above a navy pinstripe suit.

'No, Dan, but close enough after five years. Meet me for a drink sometime?' Dan thrusts a business card at me before being swallowed up in a rush for the bar.

Weeks pass, the first winter chill bites as I walk to work. I thrust my hands in my pockets to keep warm, find the card from Dan. I could phone him, make a change from being on my own tonight when Paul's on late shift. My hints for a family are wasted. We're never home together! Every evening loneliness tears me apart. This evening Paul's not due home for another two hours at leas. My hands tremble as I pick up the phone. I slip out into the starlit night to meet Dan. As promised he takes me to see his yacht.

In the moonlight the silver and blue painted yacht sparkles.

'Must be doing okay for yourself.'

'The motor trade is booming, thought I'd treat myself.'

Dan laughs, a deep booming laugh. He grips my hand tight as we step onto the yacht.

'Dreamer. That's her name. Now we can share dreams together.' He wraps a strong arm round my shoulders leading me inside. I hold the memory of those few hours of forbidden love tight. I start to look forward to Paul's late shifts.

Dan's rough hands, holding me tight, gentle rhythm of the boat rocking, starlight nights. The thrill of secret meetings, stolen, shameful, yet sheer ecstasy as the pain within is silenced.

Saturday nights I dance with Paul.

'Love you Jo' he said.

I reach for another drink to drown my guilt. The shame of lies, betrayal, broken trust, is added to a well of guilt already inside of me. Vodka numbs the bitter taste of the sin I feel at cheating on my loving husband. It doesn't even touch the well of guilt I've felt since Gran died. I should have told someone of my fears. My fear of the machines Gran was attached to, my fear of losing Gran. My terror of loneliness. I should have stopped her from dying. I reach for another drink as years of pent up emotions threaten to surface. As a child I felt anger, hurt, confusion at my mother's changing moods and tears. I learned to keep my feelings inside. I tried to be good, quiet, so that mum wouldn't get ill again.

The price of escape

During this time I seek release from feelings of guilt that haunt me. If I'd told someone I was scared, would Gran have died? If I'd been a better friend to Susan, would she have left? I should be honest, at least with myself. Paul deserves better than me. These thoughts drag me further into depression and desperation. I escape for a little while, for as long as the next drink or dance lasts. I also visit my doctor, requesting sleeping tablets, my desperate attempt to block the nightmares.

That night I dream I'm a little girl. Mummy is crying. I don't know why. She is spreading out sweeties on the kitchen table. This is a new game. I'm not usually allowed sweets until after dinner. I stand on tiptoes to reach the sweets. Mummy cries. I tug at her woollen cardigan, give her my pink teddy bear. She smiles at me through her tears. We eat the sweeties together.
A big black shadow comes in over us. The room is dark. I reach out to grab mummy's hand. She's gone. I'm alone in the dark. Someone calls out. I wake, sweating, realising I'm calling out for my mother. This same dream is repeated. Sometimes dad is there. Always I wake crying for my mother.

When alcohol fails to drown the guilt and shame, I turn again to self-injury. My life becomes a dangerous cocktail of alcohol, medication, lies and cutting. One night I curl into Paul's arms shaking in terror as the bedroom curtains become snakes. A few days later I wake in Paul's arms.
'What happened?' I mumble.
I stare into Paul's white, drawn face.
'You nearly died Jo.'
I try to lift my head, but my neck is like jelly.
'First me, then paramedics re-started your heart.'

'Sorry' I wheeze, touching my black swollen ribs, scraped arms.

'I made a mistake with my sleeping tablets.'

'Be careful Jo' Paul said, later handing me a mug of black coffee.

'I don't want to lose you.'

I resort to other methods of self-harming e.g. risk-taking, bruising, to keep my self-injury hidden. No more cutting. It seems impossible to give up. Since Gran died I've self-harmed to keep the pain of loneliness away. My self-injury is my way of communicating within myself, a release of tension as feelings build inside. Paul seems satisfied. His warmth to me grows with the longer, brighter days.

I'm not trying to kill myself, only my feeling with my self-harming, which includes alcohol, medication abuse and self-injury. To me self-injury is my lifeline, my only way to survive the pain I feel inside. I'm becoming increasingly restless as one by one my feelings of guilt and shame about Paul and Gran bubble to the surface.

The survival of self-injury

If you are actively self-injuring, remember the basics of first aid and care for your wounds.

Scars tell a silent story of inner pain and turmoil. However, not everyone is understanding or accepting. If you feel pushed away by others, especially if you feel rejected, try to care for yourself. Listen to your feelings. Would a warm bubble bath, instrumental music or prayer be comforting? Would deep breathing or relaxation techniques help you feel more in control? You can find a lot of support and information via the Internet on self-injury and related issues. My personal favourite site is siari.co.uk.

Early spring, Paul too seems restless after a winter of overtime.

'My office is supporting the local scout group to go on a day trip to Wales. Would you like to come as a helper Jo?'

It's a long day's journey. First the small rattling train and then a long hike to the top of the mountain. Tonight when the scouts are settled, I'll talk to Paul about our first baby. Far ahead I hear the scouts laughing and joking. I reach out my hand to the youngest scout trailing behind. Long lost memories of holding Gran's hand echo in the whistling wind. I remember looking up at Gran. She had her best wool coat on.

'You must be a good girl for the nice lady.'

I look up at the strange woman in the navy dress; she has a badge on her collar.

'This is Mrs Jones, she will be taking care of you with all the other children.'

I was clinging onto Gran's coat when she said goodbye.

'Don't cry' she said.

My body shakes, I'm back to reality.

Back at home, I feel trapped. With Paul home most evenings we have no overtime money. I have no excuse to go out. A gnawing longing fills me inside.

'Children?'

I cuddle up to Paul.

'It's not the right time.'

The following day Paul arrives home with a large box that appears to be squeaking.

'They're wonderful'

I fuss over the tiny kittens, two innocent balls of fluff that bring laughter, tears of joy and chaos.

'Sparky. Come back, you're not a chimney sweep!'

Too late, our bed-sit is covered with soot as Sparky does a victory run. Dusty's tricks range from swinging on curtains, to chasing bath bubbles, the latter ends in her first and only swimming lesson. Soon the kittens are piling on weight, growing into contented cats.

The miracle of life

Life continues.

The cats provide love, fun and chaos to our bed-sit. Each day when Paul arrives home, the kitchen is filled with daffodils and freshly baked bread or cakes. Even at times of great suffering there is beauty to be found in nature. In the power of crashing waves, the determination of spring bulbs bursting through frosty ground to brighten dull days.

When you are feeling depressed it is easy to feel overwhelmed, that the day looms ahead as one great black mass. Try to break the day up into hours or half hours and set goals for each hour e.g. have a bath, clean your bedroom, have a walk. Remember to include rest periods e.g. coffee time, time for relaxation. Try to include activities you enjoy, or used to enjoy, perhaps listening to music, phone a friend or gardening. If you have a task to do that still feels too much, break it down into small steps:

1. Make bed
2. Tidy up magazines, papers
3. Dust
4. Hoover

Remember to reward yourself, give yourself praise for all efforts. Life is difficult when you are depressed. If you had a broken arm you would give yourself extra time and not expect so much from yourself. Depression is just as much a disability, so give yourself extra time and reward and praise every effort.

Late spring I fill our bed-sit with bluebells. One Sunday morning I'm preparing lunch when the phone rings.

'Aunt Betty's in hospital, possible break, fall'

I rush round the bed-sit after reassuring my mother, as if I can stop the screaming in my head by keeping busy.

'That's your aunt's third fall recently' Paul comments later.

'It's happening again, everyone will leave or die.'

'Don't be silly. People move on. You're not alone. You've got me and two cats.'

In the weeks that follow I throw myself into work, Annie isn't replaced. Most days I return home exhausted, Paul dozes on the settee, our nights out stop. I still secretly mix medication and alcohol, falling deeper into my own private hell. On our occasional nights out, friends question Paul.

'Jo's changed, is anything wrong?'

'What happened to her arms?'

'I fight tigers'

I laugh, joke, anything to stop the questions. I dread questions, others may learn I'm bad. Bad girls cry. Bad children go to hell. The unspoken, yet clear message from my mother, she was ill at the time. Bad girls cry, bad children go to hell. I must be good, quiet, not ask questions. Keep my terrible secret. I was a bad child. I was so bad mummy got ill. They took my mummy away. If ever I was bad again, maybe they would come back? I'd be alone, I'd be to blame. Thankfully, now I know these thoughts and fears are untrue.

I'm now a regular visitor at the local hospital. Cowering in a worn duffle coat, I peer at staff through a haze of alcohol.

'Why?'

'You're young. Married even.'

'Go away. Do a proper job.'

One Friday night, the full moon lights up a body slumped on a bench in the village square. Tatty old duffle coat, broken bottle dangling, pools of vomit lie beneath me.

'What happened love?'

I look up into the policeman's dark eyes.

'Hurt me… cold… left me alone…'

I want to explain I've been raped. I want someone to care, words stick in my throat. Most of all, I want a bath, to scrub soak off this feeling of evil that has filled me. I feel filthy, disgusting, used. My body has been taken, abused and cast aside like an empty beer can. I tense as the policeman helps me to my feet.

'You should go to hospital.'

'No, I need to go home.'

Later, at home I scrub my skin until it's raw, trying to clean away the badness.

The following evening I'm at A&E, I've self-injured again in an attempt to cleanse myself, as well as to draw boundaries between the man who raped me, and myself. Tight bandages, security in routine, I look up as the curtains are swept aside.

'Paul?'

'Doctor Smith, duty psychiatrist, time we had a chat isn't it Jo?'

'Someone's following me. They're going to kill me. I'm scared. Will you help?'

The doctor sits, leans forward patiently takes notes. After some time he folds his papers.

'I think you should attend the psychiatric day centre between shifts at work.'

Who am I? What am I? Where am I?

At this time, due to shutting out all feelings, I'm not sure who I am anymore. My fighting spirit remains though.

I remember as a child, long nights rocking in pain. I was too scared to cry. I learned to dream. Breathing in short shallow breaths, I'd imagine beautiful snow-capped mountains overlooking clear blue lakes. In my dream my dad would hug me, in his arms I'd be safe. Dad would take away the pain I felt inside.

My self-injury becomes my way of communication. Often misinterpreted by others, maybe they're scared?

The first weeks I spend at the day centre, I say 'I'm okay.' I refuse to let anyone close enough to see the pain and guilt I feel inside, at my strange secret life. On the outside I work hard, care for my husband and two cats, visit my parents.

My secret life is different. I live two separate lives, one 'normal' life, one a mix of stolen hours of love, medication and alcohol. I learned as a child to shut out painful events. I listened to mummy, yet I shut out my feelings. Mummy cried, I listened. I tried to be good. The damage of my self-injury increases as I close more and more into my own private world. I have since learned this is called dissociation from reality.

Due to time off sick I've lost my job. My old friend self-injury calls again. This time it's different. I must die. The summer sun beats down outside, inside I feel cold and lifeless. Outside I hear children laughing, inside I scream out in pain. I want to kill my feelings. I want to die. I fight these thoughts of death as I clean our bed-sit and change the bedding. The cats run from the bedroom as I hoover.

'I must be strong, I have to care for you.'

Sparky rubs his head against my legs as if in answer.

'Paul can care for you. He doesn't need me. I'm just a burden.'

Voices scream inside my head. 'You're bad. Bad girls cry.' My thoughts explode into a mass of destruction. There is only one way out... to die.

I want to be with Gran, she's the only one who ever understood. Gran never asked questions, she just hugged me. We would talk over cups of tea and shortbread biscuits.

I don't deserve to be with Paul, I'm hurting him with my self-injury, lies and deceit. I've lost my job. My whole life is a mess.

I lock the backdoor. I turn the stereo up to maximum volume. No work, no friends, even the doctor was hopeless. He didn't care for me as my dad used to.

As a young child when I had nightmares sometimes dad would come when I cried. He would hold me in his arms. His towelling dressing gown was soft to cuddle up to. Dad would read me stories until the nightmares and demons promised to go away.

I sink to the bathroom floor. Red tears flow. Outside the sun beats down. I hear our neighbours clattering round his roof garden. I try to call out. 'No more lonely nights' plays on the stereo as I slump unconscious.

Days later Paul tells me how he climbed over the roof and then broke into the bed-sit to get help for me. He risked his life for me.

Much as I hate being trapped in hospital there is security in the routine of a psychiatric ward. Night time is the best time. One of the staff, Tony, runs a small art therapy group.

The first night I splash black and red paint across the paper. Pain, loneliness, despair, shattered dreams flood out. Paper becomes a substitute for my arms. With Tony's patient encouragement I start to talk a little.

The benefits of art therapy.
This is from a self-injurer's perspective. For a professional perspective please see references at the end of this book.

1. To communicate, without the need to find words.
2. To draw boundaries between others and myself. In order to maintain a sense of self, we need to be clear about what we feel and what others feel.
3. To feel listened to and accepted.
4. Art became a way for me to express my 'unsafe' feelings of pain, anger and rejection.
5. Art is a safe place for the voices to be heard
6. Art is a way of searching for and finding answers to problems
7. Art can be a release, as pent up feelings are expressed on paper.

You have choices to make over what materials to use, whether to use colour or black and white, to use structure or plain drawings. In art therapy you can use clear portraits or abstract words, letters, numbers, symbols or poetry. This gives the mind freedom to explore the problem without the threat of feeling judged or misunderstood. The piece of artwork you do is yours. You decide how much to share about what your picture means.

I value talking, sharing with others. We listen, empathise, show care and support for each other. Sometimes others see elements in my picture I didn't know were there. Elements of pain I put on paper unconsciously, because I was relaxed. Putting the broken pieces of my life and feelings onto paper is a healing process. Once these pieces are on paper you can see what is missing. Other group members help to identify parts; slowly it is possible to piece the broken bits together.

I talk a little at the centre but still feel unable to own my feelings. After a few months I find temporary work at a factory.

One week to Christmas and, once again, I find myself without work. Unable to face Paul, to argue again if we buy food or coal for the fire, I head for the chemist shop. White glistening snow, marked only by cat paw prints is tinged pink as I enter our bed-sit. I couldn't even wait to get home. In desperation I tear at my arms.

Back in hospital again, Christmas eve, I ask to see my doctor.
'Can I go home for Christmas?'
'Yes. I'll also be putting in a referral for you to see someone else.'

'No...please...' I stutter. 'I'm starting to trust you a little.' For the first time I start to share my fears...

Trust me...

Trust takes time to build. Start by taking small risks. Tell the person you are working with your feelings. Start with one problem you feel you can share. Try writing a list of problems and then pick the one you choose to talk about. If it is difficult to find words, maybe you could share writing, poems or artwork.

The New Year is a fresh start for me. I find work at a small catering firm on the outskirts of the village. Jack, the driver, shares his lukewarm coffee from his thermos flask with me.

'You been here long?' I ask.

'Stick with me, I'll see you're okay.'

Jack breaks his sandwiches in half to share too.

Over the winter months we become allays against the penny-pinching boss.

In the cold freeze of February Jack confides in me.

'I never even get a hug at home. It's lonely you know.'

Touched by Jack's pain I reach up and kiss Jack by his ear.

'Goodnight my friend.'

The next evening Jack leads me up the rickety staircase to the storerooms.

'Something to show you.' I back against the cold stone wall, desperate to escape his strong hands. Hot panting breath, hands of steel, desperation burns in Jack's eyes.

'Don't tell. I need you. You're my friend remember?'

'You're late tonight,' Paul greets me. 'The stew I made burnt.'

'The cats can have the burnt bits.' I pick up two fluffy bundles, their warmth and purrs soothe the pain I feel inside.

'We could start a family, now we're both working.'

'There's plenty time, besides we haven't got the money for you to give up work.' Paul always has ready excuses.

During my late evenings with Jack, my boss, pain, shame, guilt is my only gain.

'Here's a bottle of Rum for your Paul's birthday.'

So that's all I'm worth now, a cheap brand name bottle of spirits. Blinded by anger, guilt, shame, I run to my secret friend. I hate myself at this time. I feel disgusted with my body, I feel dirty and used. Yet I carry on with this arrangement with Jack as I think of him as my only friend. Months pass, my self-esteem keeps falling.

Looking at the benefits of communication versus the secret language of self-injury

Advantages of self-injury: personal, private, mine, time out, artistic, expression, sexual, cleansing, release, calming, exhilarating, exciting.
Negatives of self-injury: misunderstood, painful, rejecting, isolating, loss of respect, loss of self esteem, no negotiation, punished, work problems, scars, long term physical damage, loss of friends.

Advantages of communication, either talking, writing or art: direct, open, honesty, caring, considerate, shared pain, acceptance, company, increased respect, increased self-esteem, loving, improved work relations, equality, negotiation, release, calming, exciting.

My aunt has several more falls.
'Clumsy, icy roads, missed my footing.'
My aunt Betty has nearly as many excuses as me. Her grace and determination shine to the last, against the mystery illness that has even the specialists baffled. I visit occasionally. My aunt is in hospital now. As I take her hand, she cries. Tears run rivers down her grey face. I stand.
'Goodbye. I'll be back soon.' I never return. The pain of remembering Gran like this is too much to bear. I add guilt at leaving my aunt to the guilt I felt when Gran died.

Spring flowers burst open. I see them in a blur. Jack has been taken ill so I've taken on his duties. I race round in the battered works van, radio blaring. My 'prize' for being good, Jack taught me to drive. The van squeals, rocks, I take corners at fifty miles per hour, throw sacks of potatoes into steaming kitchens. I have little time to think with working between sixty and seventy hours a week.

'You've been working hard, how about a break?' Paul asks.
'Jack's back next week.'
'Kirsty and Phillip from scouts have booked a self-catering cottage in the Lake District.'
'What are we waiting for?' I laugh as I hand Paul the phone.

Our rucksacks are packed. The cat's food and keys are with our neighbour. Paul shouts, 'Hurry up, we'll miss the train.'
I'm locking the door as the phone rings.
'Jo it's mum... Aunt Betty died at six o'clock this morning...'
Four days later, Kirsty, Philip and Paul are sitting on top of the green hill, breaking open a picnic lunch. I wander off quietly. Looking down at the sheer drop I shed a silent tear for Aunt Betty, for Gran for myself.
'Goodbye Gran.'

- If you are having difficulty with emotional memories or flashbacks, please seek professional help. Initially self-injury may seem to be a necessary coping strategy but remember you are worth more.
- If you are a harsh judge of yourself, try to see how others see you. Do they really hate you as much as you hate yourself? People show love, even in our darkest moments. A gentleman called an ambulance, knelt in mud ignoring his new pinstripe suit. He stayed with the vomit and blood soaked teenager. I never knew his name... thank you for staying, for caring.
- Just once, can you try to be kind to yourself instead of self-harming?
- There is no failure. Only learning experiences. Even through my lowest points a tiny spark of love keeps me fighting. You are worth fighting for too. There is hope.

Crisis coping tips:
- Phone a friend.

- Cry. It really does help release tension.
- Play the reality game.
- Write down feelings.
- Exercise.

<u>Dancing in pools of moonlight</u>

   Sunday afternoon, Paul and me arrive with bags bursting with gifts. My dad grins as he unwraps bottles of beer and souvenir packets of sweets.
   'Thanks Jo, Paul.'
   Mother paces, wrings her hands.
   'Jo, aunt Betty… she left you some money.'
   Paul is first to break the awkward silence.
   'That's great news. Let's go home and unpack.'
   Weeks pass, I bank my cheque. I should be happy, yet nightmares return. One night I wake screaming.
   'What is it?' Paul reaches out, holds me. Between racking sobs I explain.
   'I left aunt Betty alone. I left Gran to die. I'm bad. I don't deserve the money.'
   'Don't be silly.' Paul ruffles my hair. 'We can have a proper holiday, Philip and Kirsty are going to Austria.'
   'I'd love to see the mountains.'

   First week in January, we're boarding the plane to Austria.

Chapter Three

The Pain of Our Inner Child

Dancing in pools of moonlight

Sunday afternoon I arrive back home with Paul, bags bursting with gifts. Jeff, my dad, grins as he unwraps bottles of beer and packets of Kendal mint cake.

'Thanks Jo, Paul.'

Mother seems restless, she shuffles, wrings her hands.

'Jo, Aunt Betty…she left you some money.'

Paul is the first to break the awkward silence filling the tiny lounge.

'That's great news. Now let's get home and unpack.'

Weeks pass, long sleepless nights, nightmares return. By day, haunting memories of leaving Aunt Betty alone. I left her alone…crying.

One night I wake screaming.

'What is it?' Paul reaches out, holds me.

'I'm bad. I don't deserve this money.'

'Your aunt Betty never had children, she thought a lot of you Jo. Tell me in the morning what you want to do.'

Six o'clock I shake Paul awake. 'I'm handing in my notice at work.'

'You haven't got that much money silly.'

'No, but I've enough for a week or two until I get another job.

Ten days later I start work at the local supermarket, we arrange a party for the weekend. Following generous measures of Paul's homemade punch only myself, Paul, Kristy and Phillip are left to send out for a Chinese take-out.

'We're off to Austria for a skiing holiday in the New Year, would you two like to join us?' Phillip asks.

I remember as a child, waiting at my bedroom window for my dad to come home. I wanted us to escape far away to lakes and mountains like in my fairytale book.

Mid January, with Phillip and Kristy, we head off to Austria. Paul is a natural, takes to skiing as if skis are extensions of his legs. He glides effortlessly across the ski slopes.

'Come on Jo, keep up.' Paul laughs as Phillip hauls a tangled mass of skis and sticks out of another hole. Lunchtime we relax with mugs of steaming hot chocolate in our favourite lakeside café.

'There's a coach trip this afternoon, across the mountains to the next village.'

'Let's go,' I say, 'I need an easy way to the top of these mountains.'

At the top of the snow-capped mountain, the coach stops for photographs.

'I'll remember this moment forever,' I said, hugging Paul.

'Me too. You're standing on my toes!' Looking out over the lakes and mountains I feel total peace. The village below is like a child's toy set.

Perspective

It is useful to get a different perspective on life events, although we do not have to travel away from home in order to achieve this. What can be helpful is to talk things through with a friend, or to go for a long walk, somewhere quiet. In our increasingly busy world, silence and space can be difficult to find. I've found the silence and natural spaces of woodland, parks, the sea shore healing. Take time out from a busy schedule to spend away from the hustle and bustle. Take a walk, learn to appreciate nature. Take time for you, to note and feel your feelings... before they become overwhelming. When you feel that you could explode, can't take anymore, have to self-harm... STOP! Find an alternative...

- Write down feelings, words, ideas
- Talk with someone you trust
- Have a walk
- Listen to music
- Try art, craft, knitting, sewing
- Sit with feelings... they will pass
- Make a jigsaw puzzle

- Take a shower or bath

If you have self-harmed, remember you're not a failure or useless, it's not a disaster. You don't need to be perfect... no one is! Be kind to yourself, gently ask what can I learn from this experience?

During my time on holiday, I decide to talk with Jack, to make peace with him on my return home.

Walking home after my first day back at work I pick up a copy of the local paper.

'Man found on beach, two days ago identified as local man Jack Fothergill.'

The headlines scream at me long after I've used the paper to light the fire at home. I think of cutting as flames lick up the chimney. I haven't cut for at least two months now. Voices still taunt me, beckoning from my memories. I wonder when the next time will be.... Know it has to be right. My secret ritual is developing, the voices more demanding. My self-injury is less impulsive, though at times the damage is more severe.

<u>The ritual of self-injury</u>

With the development of my self-injury, the addictive nature starts to show. I need to do more damage to get the same relief. My self-injury fast becomes my coping mechanism. Automatic reflex. Pain, cut, rejection, guilt, pain. In desperation I seek relief in alcohol, abuse medication. I take risks, often paying dearly. Confusion, screaming voices grow in my head; due to my not acknowledging or allowing feelings. The more I self-injured the deeper I fall into despair. My risk-taking increases. Raped and sexually abused, long nights screaming inside.

Only now, looking back I see patterns to my life events and feelings. When I was raped and abused I felt at rock bottom. My self-esteem was zero. I survived in hate. I hated my body, my life, and the world in general. It was only when I started to respect and care for myself that others started to respect me. I reached rock bottom before I discovered this. Each day that passes remind yourself you are special, unique, worthwhile.

Challenge negative thoughts… because one thing has gone wrong doesn't mean your whole life is bad. Keep calm, be cool! Take a break, think things through.

I attend Jack's funeral, sadness, guilt, relief and anger wash over me in veils of tears. 'Jack, my friend, you cared for me. You used me too.' I whisper as I leave the church.

Back at work, I grab a quick coffee with my friend Angela.

'I'm going to drama club tonight, why not join me? You look like you need cheering up.'

My curiosity at seeing quiet, shy Angela on stage leads me to join the group. Evenings fill with fun and laughter as we make props, paint backdrops, learn lines. Acting provides a welcome relief from arguments at home. Paul and me still have opposing views on starting a family.

Communication

For anyone struggling with self-injury, communication is difficult. For me my scars became my way of silent speech. My wounds cried silently for me. Self-injury became my secret language of hurt and shame, a way of both punishing and comforting myself. There are alternatives. In drama, through acting out another role, we may find unknown confidence and a way of expressing feelings in a safe way. Music, both to learn to play a musical instrument or listen to a favourite piece of music can calm the urges to self-harm. Art, to splash colours, inks, to make a collage, all these can express feelings. You don't need to be an artist to express feelings.
Try walking somewhere quiet, maybe a local park, or nature walk.

If you have self-injured remember to take care of yourself physically, basic first aid. If necessary attend the A&E department of your local hospital. If this is daunting, take a friend for support.

Next remember your emotional needs. Do you need comfort, calm, or to feel in control? For comfort try wearing or stroking, a favourite woollen jumper. Make a fuss of your pets if you have any. Have a mug of tea. Calming activities, relaxation breathing, count to ten slowly, play instrumental music.

To feel more in control play the reality game:
- Name five things you can see
- Name four things you can hear
- Name three things you can feel
- Name two things you can smell (or like the smell of)
- Name one thing you like about yourself.

I found this game on the Internet a couple of years ago and it really does work. You could also phone a friend, or the Samaritans.

Try to go with your own feelings and needs, do whatever you need to that is comforting and safe.

The first autumn leaves fall. On my way to drama club, I scuff piles of leaves. Remembering myself as a child bouncing happily in the garden. 'Daddy look!'

'I've only just raked those.' Dad is laughing as he hugs me, pulling leaves from my hair. I've found happy memories of a child still alive within.

Weeks later, a television programme is launched. 'Protect our children from abuse.'

'Many children suffer abuse, of different kinds. Physical, sexual, emotional, we want to help those children. The television presenter seems to be talking directly to me.

I'm beginning to identify the screams in my head as those of my inner child, hurt, screaming in pain. Never accepted or understood. I was a child old beyond her years.

'When I hurt now, it's like I'm a child, hurting again. That's why I cut, to stop the screaming.' I'm trying to explain this new idea to myself as much as to Paul.

'Did your parents hurt you?' Paul asks.

'Not deliberately, but mum was ill. She was very ill for a long time. There was only me for her to talk to. I didn't always understand, I just knew mummy hurt and I couldn't make her pain go away.'

Over the next few weeks memories haunt me. Voices scream in my head. 'You're bad. Guilty. Shameful. To break secrets is bad. I'm feeling eaten up with guilt, as my parents never deliberately hurt me. My mother was suffering from chronic depression and turned to me as her only support.

I try my best to cope. I throw myself into work, keep the house clean and tidy, and care for Paul. Most evenings I curl up close to Paul, clinging to him as my rock, my safe place. Memories still haunt me, I turn to cutting again.

<u>Dealing with memories and flashbacks</u>

When you are troubled by painful memories or flashbacks it is important to be kind to yourself. Try to ground yourself in the reality of today. Place your feet firmly on the floor. Remember that although the memories may be painful, they are a part of your past and can't hurt you anymore. Take things slowly, one day, one hour at a time. Focus on one job at a time. Try relaxation, deep breathing, play calming music, whatever works for you. I've found feelings of anger particularly hard to deal with. Try crying, or screaming, into a pillow or thumping cushions or pillows. Play sport or have a walk. You could join a martial arts class. Find somewhere quiet and scream or join an assertiveness training course to learn to channel anger in positive ways.

You could also write a letter to the person who hurt you... this one is not for posting so you can say exactly what's on your mind.

One Friday afternoon, mid winter, the supermarket is quiet.
'You're owed time Jo, have a half day.'

I waste no time, grab my coat, run home. Great, I'll tidy, get tea ready, light the fire, have the lounge all cosy for when Paul gets home from work. We'll talk about children. I'm forever optimistic.

I drop the oven tray as the door slams.

'You're home early! Leave that. Tea can wait. I've something to tell you.' I try to stand firm, my body shakes at Paul's unusually harsh voice.

36

'I'm leaving. Found someone else. Can't take any more of you.' I grab the armchair as the room spins wildly, fight to regain control. There are no words, even if I could find a voice.

The first weeks of being alone I clean the bed-sit every day. Every evening I put out Paul's mug of tea. Reality hits hard. I'm alone. Waking at two o'clock struggling to make sense of the pile of bills and bank statements. Long nights, half-eaten pot noodles, my only solace finishing the dregs from the drinks cabinet.
Paul seems anxious to start his new life. 'Sign these papers Jo. I need a quick divorce.'
'I'll meet you for a drink Friday. I'll bring the papers.'
Friday evening I step out in my neatly pressed skirt and blouse. I'm full of confidence as I fling open the pub door and wave to Paul.
'So you must be Janice'
'Jo, you know this is Maria'
'Excuse us. We need to talk' I grab Paul's arm, my great plan's breaking as my eyes fill.
'Paul, please come back. I'm sorry.'
'It's too late Jo. Maria is expecting our baby. I'm so pleased, so proud to be a father to Maria's baby.'
'I hate that woman. You never wanted my baby. How could you?' I fight back tears as I run from the pub.

Reaching deep within I find the strength to keep our bed-sit going. To keep the bills paid and, to forget the pain, I feel I throw myself into work. One busy Friday the store man is off sick. 'It's okay. I'll unload the crates.'
'Jo, those crates are heavy.'
'It's too late.' I cry as the top crate slips, crashing down, breaking, tearing my right arm.
Lonely nights, no-one sees my tears. No-one hears my silent screams. The pain is deep, emotional pain throbs with my arm, in plaster now. Memories echo in my mind. In desperate nights a little girl crying, her tiny body twisted in agony. 'Milk allergy.' Doctors announced after months of invasive tests and surgery. Don't let them see you cry. Be good, be quiet. Flashbacks that

make no sense, 'sweets, eat the sweeties.' Mummy was crying. Be a good girl, don't cry.

I pace the floor, clutching my arm. I feel abandoned. I feel like a child again. Alone, I stare out at the night sky, look at the stars and think of Gran.

Memories of comfort

I hope that like me, you have at least one comforting memory to hold. Throughout my childhood my Gran held my life together. Gran's warm hugs, welcoming smile, teapot and biscuits always ready for friends and strangers alike. Gran's unconditional love held me safe. I was seventeen when Gran died. I tried to control my feelings, but after leaving home seventeen years of pent up emotion exploded into self-injury.

Looking back, I see that a number of events contributed to my choice to survive by self-injury.

As a child my mother was seriously ill. I was separated from my family for three months, in a large building with many other children: the 1960s children's home. As an adult, I understand, it's too frightening for a child to see parents or carers as unable to cope. It's easier for the child to see herself as 'bad'. I also learned from an early age to keep my feelings inside. These feelings remained trapped inside of me. My fear of mother leaving. My insecurity, hurt and shame at being a bad girl. I kept all these feelings inside. As an adult I identify these feelings as my hurt inner child. This void of pain and despair is my inner child. As I feel ashamed to admit my feelings, even to myself, I turn to self-injury to stop myself feeling. My self-injury both punishes and soothes my inner child.

Spring bursts with new hope, my arm is recovering, and I'm back at work. My dad is taken ill, rushed into hospital with a heart attack. I still remain optimistic. Dad is a great fighter and seems to regain his strength quickly. Wednesday evenings are still the highlights of my week; I meet Judy at the drama club. On stage I transform easily into outrageous characters.

'How do you do it?'

'I forget I'm scared.'

I wish I could forget the loneliness that sweeps over me back at the bed-sit. One Saturday evening I pluck up courage to phone Dan.

'I'm too busy. In the middle of a big deal.'

'Dan remember the good times...'

'You were a temporary distraction from boredom.'

'Dan I loved...' I listen to the empty dialling tone.

Feeling my last hope of comfort has been crushed I turn to my old friend self-injury again.

Is it possible to change?

Yes, change is always possible. Breaking free from self-injury is life enhancing, involving changes at every level. We can also choose to see events differently. Although I couldn't see it at the time, breaking my arm was a positive learning experience. It took months for my arm to heal. I had to write, draw and even eat with my left hand only. Through painting left-handed I found my art style developing and changing. Freestyle, abstract, less restricted than my pen and ink drawings. My former paintings were delicate, intricate, controlled, painfully controlled. Black ink, white paper; stark images of good and bad. I'm finding my new style of painting a useful way to let my feelings out.

Instead of seeing change as being threatening we can choose to see it as a challenge. Start with small daily changes. Begin to love yourself, believe in yourself. It is possible to break free from self-injury, one day at a time. Think of one positive thought about yourself each day to build your self esteem.

Naming the void inside

I can now name the void of pain I feel inside as my inner child crying. At this time I feel unable to share my thoughts and feelings with anyone. This is my deep dark secret of guilt that I'm ashamed to own even to myself.

Owning our feelings, such as 'I feel angry,' 'I feel hurt,' is a step towards taking control in a positive way. It's normal to have feelings. There are no right or wrong feelings, only uncomfortable feelings that we can learn to live through with acceptance and love. Try to take care of yourself as a whole person. (I know this is difficult!) Remember that body, mind and spirit all need loving care. Take even one small step, healthy eating plan, exercise, or try relaxation. Remember one small step at a time is all that is needed.

Crisis coping tips:

- Art - try using paint and paper rather than self-injury to express feelings
- Take time out - remember today's pain will ease, feelings will pass
- Read or write poetry
- Try to let others closer - when we feel hurt it is natural to push others away, yet that's when our need for support is greatest.

Chapter Four

Dawn Breaks, I Hide Away in Shame

Three weeks to Christmas, the village supermarket bustles with shoppers. Tills ring, competing with piped music and screaming children.

'Time you filled the biscuits Jo.'

'Don't forget you're on tills in ten minutes.'

I rub my arm, though the break healed, the pain burns after lifting.

'Jo, phone for you, be quick,' the supervisor sighs. 'It's difficult enough keeping all the tills open without personal phone calls.'

'Jo, it's Mum. Your Dad's had another mild heart attack. He's resting now. Can you call in on your way home with milk?'

I rest my head against the cold office wall, trying to stop the screaming. It never stops. Constant demands at work, lonely nights, and dad ill. Memories of Dan, love and loss, bittersweet memories of Jack, love at any cost.

'You okay Jo?' The supervisor pulls a chair out as I feel my legs crumple.

'My dad's had a heart attack. I need to...'

'Go home. See your dad, I'll cover somehow. We'll need you in at seven o'clock tomorrow. Get an early night Jo, you look exhausted.'

I have an urgent appointment with the voices in my head. I run to the chemist, blades, cleansed, I'm free. Time stops, the screaming ends. My self-injury is impulsive, frightening, it is also necessary to my survival. During the time I self-injure I talk to the voices in my head, pleading for freedom. I plead with the judge to stop the cutting. Only when the judge is satisfied can I stop. Only when the voices are silent am I free. The release, expression of emotion is complete. I feel totally calm and peaceful. The world is a beautiful place.

Choices

Do I have a choice? At times of great stress it's easy to forget we have choices. If you find yourself under stress, please STOP!

Slow enough to make a choice between self-harm and healthier choices. Maybe you can phone a friend, or write how you feel, or use distractions.

When we are under pressure, we often choose a familiar way, even if it's unhealthy. I'm turning to self-injury to express my feelings. My self-injury is comforting in its familiarity, also punishing in its severity. My self-harm expresses the anger I feel. Anger beats out a red hot orchestra of survival, keep away, no entry... detonate! Anger hides my pain, inside I'm screaming in pain. Evil, that's me. I believe my feelings will contaminate, even destroy, anyone I let close, so I tell people keep away.

My key nurse said, 'I'm strong, I will listen. I will stay. Feelings are comfortable or uncomfortable; they are normal, not destructive or evil. Having destructive thoughts does not make you a bad person. A bad act does not make you a bad person. You are a worthwhile person who made a mistake or did one bad act.'

Red petals

Tormented by pain, both night and day...
On a bed of red petals I did lay.
Cold, dark and lonely, yet I heard you say...
Talk to me, I'll hold you, yes I will stay.

This time I found myself at the local A&E department still dissociated from reality. I pace between plastic chairs, thumb last year's magazines. I remember my mother's phone call.

'Mum, I'm sorry.' How can I explain the desperation that drives me to cut?

'Why Jo?'

'I just...

'You've let us down, again. It's nine o'clock. I've been phoning around, searching for you.'

'I'll be there soon.'

'Stay there. The ambulance is coming. You're killing your father with all this worry.'

Coronary care unit: silence is broken only by the low hum of machines.

'Only five minutes and be quiet.' Ward sister stands at the door like a watchman on guard duty. I clasp my dad's clammy hand.

'Dad,' I whisper, 'it's okay. I'll take care of you.' I catch faint familiar smell of Old Spice. For a moment I'm a little girl.

Remembering being curled up in daddy's arms. Daddy felt safe, familiar smell of aftershave, soft towelling dressing gown. Daddy always made the nightmares go away.

I tuck dad's blanket closer. Dad looks up, his face pinched, white. A single tear falls to his pillow as I'm beckoned to leave.

Later that week I visit Doctor Smith, my psychiatrist.

'I think it's time you came back to group therapy Jo.'

'I don't have time. I'm working.'

'I'm running an evening group. I'll see you tonight.'

The first two weeks at the group I sit silently. The third week Doctor Smith challenges me. 'I'm sure you have something to say on tonight's discussion of love and loss Jo.'

'I still miss my Gran. I'm hurt now. Sometimes I think the hurt will never go away.'

Time heals

It is true that time heals broken hearts. It is also important to acknowledge and own our feelings. There is no easy answer to grief, but I've found talking helps. You could also make a scrapbook of memories, photos, pictures, poems, and dried flowers. These things may help express and heal the hurt you feel inside. Maybe visiting a place you shared with your loved one will help you come to terms with their loss. Whatever is best for you. The important thing is to express feelings and not keep them bottled up. I've found that keeping feelings locked up inside is a strong trigger to self-injury. The pressure of keeping feelings in inevitably grows until something has to give.

As the weeks pass I find myself looking forward to the evening group. Sharing with others seems to ease the pain I feel inside.

Christmas eve, I run home from work, as I throw my bags on the table the phone rings.

'Jo, I'm home.'

'Dad?' I hold the phone tighter, wheezing whistles in my ear.

'The doctor's let me home for Christmas.'

'I'll be round in the morning then with your presents.'

'Mum says stay for lunch.'

Christmas day, seeing my dad's eyes sparkle as he unwraps his gifts is the best gift I could have.

The gift of love

As a child, my parents gave me the precious gift of love. They taught me how to love, to reach out to others in need. Being broke, financially and frequently physically and emotionally never stopped my parents, Verity and Jeff, helping others.

Verity held tabletop sales in her tiny lounge, to raise funds for handicapped people. Stray cats were taken in and lovingly nursed back to health. Neighbours and friends often found parcels of home-baked cakes and bread. In all situations I learned to be thankful and to give generously.

New year, I'm back at work and the evening group after the Christmas break.

'This is David. It's his first evening.'

At mid evening break, I make David a coffee. 'It gets easier.' I try to reassure David. He paces, his dark eyes darting, reflecting my insecurity.

'I've given up hope. I've been rejected so many times.'

I look longingly after David as he turns away. His lean muscular body hides a hurting little person inside.

'I know what it's like to hurt. I'm lonely too.' I confide in David the next time we meet.

'One day…' David turns away again, leaving me wondering if my gestures of friendship are wanted.

I worry about my Dad's health too, although improved he still gets pain after walking. One morning I'm waiting with my mother for Dad to get ready to go out. I sip my third coffee. 'Dad okay?'

'Be patient, he's still not well.'

'I'm sorry.'

'Why?'

'For everything, since I was little I've been trouble.'

'It wasn't your fault I was ill.' Mother looks past me… 'A lot of things went wrong before you were born.' I've waited years to hear those words from my mother, yet they're hard to accept.

Spring seems to lift David's mood. 'I've been busy in my garden, would you like to come around to see?'

'We could visit the garden centre too.'

We spend more time together, woodland walks, running into icy seawater at the beach.

Overlooking the beach are the remains of a Roman castle.

'Race you to the castle.' David shouts. High up on the headland, we cuddle up against the ruins.

'When I'm rich, I'll buy you a castle,' I said.

'You will be my princess.'

I laugh, ruffling David's hair.

'Will you marry me?'

'You mean it?'

'Is that yes then?'

The summer passes in a haze of days out with David and packing up my belongings to move into David's home. By the time I've found a buyer for the flat only the bed and a few clothes are left.

'It's okay Sparky, I'm sure I can persuade David to take you too.' Sparky cries softly as I lift him onto my bed. When I wake in the morning Sparky is quiet and still.

'It's for the best, I've just decorated my lounge. Besides, that cat was too old to be moved.'

David's words do little to comfort me.

Weeks ago I stopped going to the evening group, to have more time with David. This evening I wish I had someone to talk to, somewhere to go, I need security.

'Come to me, hide. You're bad, evil.' Old voices scream, building to an orchestral crescendo by Sunday's full moon. Running, hiding in dark shadows I slice through layers of pain, guilt and despair.

'Help, set me free.' My wounds scream silently.

'I'm sorry. Never again.' I promise David later. I wonder if I'm clinging onto an impossible dream. I push my concerns for myself and for David aside.

I am worth fighting for?

Every day we need to choose to live, love and feel. Every day I choose to live. Try to keep a balanced view; life is not absolute good or bad. We can choose to see people as teachers; events are learning opportunities.

Although my self-injury was destructive, I found strength within to survive. Years of blocking out all feeling while 'coping' takes a lot of determination and resolve. Years later I'm now able to use this strength to explore my feelings. Now I'm learning to own and express my feelings in positive ways, through artwork, writing and gardening.

About a month before the wedding David is waiting for me as I leave work.

'Jo, I've got great news. I've got a new job, doing research abroad. I'm so excited. I'll have to get organised, lots to do, packing, visas. Jo, it's what I've always dreamed of. You can come and visit, the pay is excellent, the company even pays for families to visit.'

'Wait a minute. Where are you going?' I hang onto David's hand, my body trembling.

'Australia, it will be great, in fifteen years we can retire, rich and happy.' For the rest of the evening I listen to David's plans in stunned silence.

'Fifteen years?' I ask later.

'It'll fly by. We'll both be rich, happy and think of all the fantastic holidays we'll have.' David hugs me and pours another drink.

'You must be strong, let him go.'
'You're so lucky to have such an ambitious husband.'
'How lovely, a new start for both of you.'
Other people's words of cheery advice wash over me. Inside I feel angry, rejected. I keep my thoughts and feelings to myself.

Our wedding, Christmas and New Year pass in a blur of confetti, gifts and good luck cards for David.

A bitterly cold east wind sweeps a dusting of snow over me as I hug David goodbye.

'I have to go to work early today, it's stock-taking day.'

'Stay a while. My train's not due for another half-hour yet.'

'Good luck.' I turn away, to hide my tears.

Lonely nights, long weeks pass, waiting for phone calls and letters.

'Why did you leave?' I scream at David's photograph.

'You must be strong Jo.' Mother softens her tone, 'talk with David when he comes home at Easter.'

To me, feeling abandoned, lost, heartbroken, mixed up pain from David leaving and past memories, cutting seems the only option.

'I've always been too much trouble, bad, that's why David left. I must be evil.' I don't want to spoil the precious time I get to talk with David on these thoughts so I talk with the voices in my head.

'CUT!' They scream, 'be free form the pain for a little while.' My self-injury episodes become more severe, more frequent. The voices become more demanding. 'It has to be right. Everything in its proper place. Give to me completely, body and soul, be free.'

The few letters I've received from David are crumpled, tearstained, tucked in my coat pocket as I'm admitted to hospital.

'What will your husband think?' Staff ask me.

'Why?'

'Look at the mess you're in.' Endless questions, accusations. Sometimes the nurses have time to talk, other times they're too busy. I'm still seeking peace from the voices, too scared to voice my thoughts and feelings. 'I can't live without love, I don't believe David's coming home.'

Survival or Love?

My feelings of anger, guilt, and grief I kept inside. Looking back now I know I survived by self-injury, but at a cost. (Both the long term physical damage, also damage to relationships.)
Even at times of great pain and suffering we do still have choices, we can reach out to someone and ask for support. We can also find alternative ways to express our feelings.

If you are actively self-injuring don't panic. It shows you are surviving in the best way you can at the moment. Hopefully in time you will find other choices.

'I want to self-harm!'
'What do you need?' My key worker asks…
'I want to self-harm now!!!'
'Can you identify your need?'
'I need to cry. I feel so ashamed. I'm not allowed to cry, so I want to self-harm.'
'Why can't you cry? Just let the tears out…'
'Bad girls cry! Bad children go to hell! Now you'll leave because I'm bad!'
'I'll stay. It's okay to cry.' My key worker said.
In time you will understand that the hurting part of you is your inner child. This is particularly relevant if you have been hurt as a child. When I was three years old I was separated from my mother for three months, due to my mother's illness. Feelings of abandonment have been intense and painful for me since then.

If you have been hurt as a child, either deliberately or through illness in the family please seek professional counselling. It will take time to heal wounds that are buried deep but it is possible to feel better. You will come to see this inner child as deserving of love, rather than punishment. You will be able to choose to live and take loving care of yourself instead of surviving by self-injury.

It's a long cold winter for me, in and out of hospital. Letters from David tell of busy days working, quiet evenings in the local bar. One evening the phone ringing startles me.

'I'm coming home next week. The contract the boss expected has fallen through.' That night I walk deserted streets alone, unsure whether David will still want to be with me. Pacing up and down the train station, last flakes of snow whip through my thin jacket, biting at recent scars.

'Jo, I'm home.'

David runs, arms outstretched, suntanned, healthy, only worry lines round his eyes express stress.

'Of course I still love you.' David reassures me time and again.

Spring passes in a melee of long hours at work. Hope pushes through like the daffodils in our garden. Hope for a fresh start.

'I've got a cash payment in lieu of the broken contract, let's take a break. We'll go to Paris.'

I hug David, too excited to speak.

Bright city lights, crowded streets, David eagerly shows me the tourist attractions. Together forever, we promise each other from the top of the Eiffel tower.

On our return home, the romance and excitement of Paris are soon lost under a pile of bills. David takes a temporary job in a packing shed. Held together by bonds of marriage and red bills we muddle through the summer. Often in the evenings David seems far away as he stares out at the setting sun.

The first Autumn leaves falling are like the last of our dreams crumpling. David has handed in his notice. So now we're living on my wages. Weeks pass by, David's sense of hopelessness increases with the grey drizzle outside. I try to ignore the empty Whisky bottles lined up to recycle.

Exhausted from work and caring for David, I decide to go to the drama group's pantomime auditions. Laughing, chatting with friends, I put on my clown mask to forget the daily dramas at home. Late evening I'm humming as I wander home.

'David, I'm home...It's me.' The house feels unnaturally quiet and still. After checking the bedroom I find David curled up in a corner of the spare room. Torn photographs and certificates lie like mud trodden confetti.

'Get out! I don't want you here.' David's eyes burn with fury.

'David, why?' I point at the empty bottle of whisky and painkillers. He shrugs.

'I'll phone a doctor.' I turn to get the phone.

'No!' David shouts. He grabs me. Together we lie in a tangled heap. We shuffle back from each other, staring blankly. Not recognising the other as the one we chose to love.

Hours pass, the clock strikes each painful moment by. No words, wild eyes fill... speaking volumes.

One o'clock, David sighs as his body relaxes. I run to the phone. Dawn breaks, David is in hospital. I'm heartbroken. In desperation I hide away in shame.

<u>Summary</u>

- Choosing to take responsibility - daily we choose to take responsibility for our actions as adults. As children we may have had little choice over what happened. As an adult we can choose another way through a problem rather than turn to self-injury.
- Making goals - in order to take control of our lives making daily goals can be really helpful. Try to make these goals realistic and achievable. To achieve one small goal a day will really boost your self-esteem.
- Try to extend the time between the thought or urge to self-injure and the act of injury. Begin to use distractions to lengthen the time you have to make a healthier choice. In time self-injury will become a choice rather than a necessary tool of survival.

Chapter Five

<u>My Secret Friend Beckons from the Shadows</u>

'You coming home for Christmas?' I shudder as I touch David's stone shoulder; I remember Paul asking me the same question. We're sitting on the same plastic chairs in the visiting room. The Christmas tree with one string of lights looks the same too.

David shows little interest in Christmas, gifts are opened reluctantly and piled in the kitchen. I fill our home with friends, music and food yet David still seems withdrawn.

January, the snow turns to grey slush, our days are brighter, David has a new part-time job. With my newfound hope, I decide the time has come for me to help others who struggle with self-injury. For a few weeks I keep my thoughts to myself, then I tell my mother.

'I'm going to set up a group for people like me.'

'What sort of group Jo?'

'I'm going to help others. I know what it's like to feel alone. I've felt strange, the only crazy person who self-injures. I want to help others so they don't feel alone.'

'Will you be okay? Keep yourself safe?'

With support from friends and a lot of time visiting the nursing library and making phone calls I'm learning about self-injury. I find there are national help lines and support groups available. Research is painfully slow and frustrating, the first time I try to order a book on self-injury from my local bookstore the assistant looks horrified. Through talking with my family and friends a little, I'm moving from my dark secret life to openess and hope for the future.

<u>Sharing and caring</u>

Due to the very nature of self-injury it is a secretive problem. Often the self-injurer feels alone and isolated in a seemingly uncaring world. There are people who care. Maybe you could start by trusting one person. Start to tell one person about your self-injury. Yes, this is scary, but until we let others in how can they support us and help us to heal?

It is also important to see your life as a whole, to take a holistic approach. Start from basics, are you living in a safe place? Do you have adequate food, clothing etc. If not can you get support from social services or charities?

Try to reach out to others, to make friends. Join a gym, social club, church or even just chat with people you meet daily, shopkeeper, bus driver, postman, at least you are making contact.

Two months pass, my piles of papers and books have taken over half the spare room, I feel ready to start a group.

'I'm pleased to see you well Jo, but will you cope with caring for others?' David asks.

'I'm fine. This group is something I have to do. I spent years feeling isolated. I've had to lie and hide my scars for fear of what people think. I want others to know they have hope and understanding.

The first meeting is planned for Friday evening in the village hall. I take a half-day to prepare. Tea, coffee, notes, leaflets and posters are packed in cardboard boxes, filling the hall at home. Having been free form self-injury for nearly a year I'm surprised to feel such a strong pull from my old friend. I gather the boxes and drop them inside the hall doorway ready for the meeting.

'Think many will turn up? Bit of a peculiar thing this self injustice.'

'It's called self-injury.'

'Like I said, funny.' The caretaker takes a long drag of his cigarette. 'Hope it turns out alright.'

Dark thoughts surround me as I slink into the first evening shadows. The caretaker is opening the doors for the first arrivals as I shuffle back, arms tightly bandaged.

I stand to open the meeting.

'Thank you all for coming here this evening. I thought I was free from self-injury. I want to help others who may be struggling, as you can see I'm still having problems. This is my story and what is helping me to recover.'

'Jo, you did well.' Angela and Sadie, my friends from work hug me as I blink back tears.

After a slow start to the meetings with only two other members, I receive four phone calls in one week.

'Please come around, I need to talk.'

'I'm desperate.'

'Can you help me?'

'Talk to me.' I say, gripping the phone tighter until my body coils in knots of fear for the unknown caller who needs hospital treatment.

'Do you have to go?' David holds me as my body shakes. 'You've been out already today. You can't rescue everyone!'

'I'll only be an hour.' I can't explain to David that I still carry guilt about my mother's illness and my Gran's death. I wish I could explain that I feel driven to rescue others. That in some way by reaching out to help others I can heal the pain I feel inside. The insecure, childlike part of me cries silently. The adult part of me recognises pain in others and seeks to help in whatever way possible.

The next day at work, I'm unable to concentrate, voices scream for me to self-injure. A few hours of peace follow my secret ritual of pain and shame. In total dissociation from reality I feel nothing. Time stands still. I'm unaware of damp graffiti clad walls. Blood drips. Wounds scream. Long silent screams of pain and guilt... silence. Nothing left inside. I'm cleansed, free.

Hours later the duty doctor flashes questions at me as he stitches.

'Why?'

'You're destroying your life, why?'

Three in the morning, David hands me a mug of steaming tea. It's the first thing to penetrate my secret world...

'My arms hurt, why?' I ask.

I'm called into see the manager the next day when I return to work.

'You must sort yourself out Jo. You can't keep letting us down like this. You left without even telling anyone.'

My parents too, seem unhappy with me, following a tense Sunday lunch mother talks to me.
'We never know if you're safe or not Jo.'
'I'm okay.'
'We've enough to worry about, with your Dad's brother ill and Aunt Ann in hospital. Then there's your problems.'
David and me muddle through the first weeks of Summer. I regret the coldness between my parents and myself, yet I can't explain my need to self-injure.

It's my life!

During this time I was dealing with painful memories of Jack, my boss who abused me. I also had difficult childhood memories. This can be a difficult pattern to break: we have been hurt, so we hurt ourselves believing we deserve punishment. Remember, other people may have taken away your possessions, hurt you physically, abused you sexually or emotionally. Today you have the choice to change and break that pattern of abuse. Love heals. Love will help you see a future. Acceptance and loving ourselves gives us the strength to live day-by-day, working for a brighter tomorrow.
Making contact with our inner child

Initially this may just be sensations like stomach pains, headaches or restlessness. Try to stay with these sensations, they are feelings trying to surface. Feelings can be comfortable or uncomfortable, they are not bad. Learning to accept feelings is a step towards healing. In time you may identify stomach pains as anger. For me, tense painful shoulders indicate sadness.

Some weeks later David receives a surprise phone call.
'That would be great, we'll catch up on old times. See you at the gliding club next weekend then.'
'That was Simon.'

'Must be a good mate, you've been on the phone hours.'

'We were at university together. Lost contact when he moved house. He's invited us to visit next weekend.'

It's a hot summer day. David and me eagerly gulp luke-warm drinks during our train journey. At the gliding club, David runs over to meet Simon. Over lunch they chatter away.

'Look at the time; it's nearly two o'clock. Time to get the glider ready.' I watch as David and Simon soar overhead for what seems like hours.

'You haven't lost your touch.' Simon laughs with David as they land.

'Your turn Jo,' David said.

'No way, that thing's like a matchbox. Besides I'm scared of heights.'

'I'll let you in on my secret.' Simon whispers to me.

'Really?' I laugh with Simon, 'You're scared too?'

'It's a different world up there. If you're still scared we'll come straight back.'

I cling to the safety straps, eyes closed as we lift up into clear skies.

'What do you think Jo?' I open my eyes slowly. Fields stretch away beneath us, golden corn rustling in the light breeze.

'It's great, we can see for miles, there's home far away in the distance.'

Sunday evening, David, Simon and me are still laughing, chatting at Simon's local pub. We both hug Simon goodbye, then run to catch the last train home.

Monday morning, back to work, my supervisor Sadie bubbles with excitement.

'Jo, I've got my promotion, I move up to the office next week.'

'Well done, but don't forget your friends in the basement.' I keep my voice light, to hide the sadness I feel at even this small change.

The certainty of change

In life, one thing is certain, changes will happen. For an insecure person like myself this presents constant challenges. I'm fighting the urge to run and self-injure. If we can accept change as a part of life and try to live with an open, flexible attitude life will be easier. There is peace to be found in flowing with life rather than fighting every change.

Summer melts into Autumn. With the falling leaves I watch another of my dreams break. I'd wanted to stay close to Sadie, now she was working in another department. I feel ashamed of my feelings, longings to be close to Sadie, so I run to hide. Hours pass as I seek release with my secret rituals of self-injury.

'You promised, never again you said.' David questions my latest round of injuries.

'I tried.'

'Not hard enough.'

'I wish I could disappear.' I tell the doctor at the A&E department.

'It's time you went back to the centre. Get some help, we can't keep patching you up like this.'

First day back at the centre, I stay on the edge of the crowd, backed into a corner. I remember as a child trying to slope my shoulders, hide away. I wanted to escape the school bullies, block out my mother's words. I was running from life.

'Jo, you coming into the art group?'

I look up, 'Tony?'

'It's been a long time since I've seen you Jo. Have you still been drawing?' I don't reply, I sit silently. My tears mingle with dark shadows as I put my feelings onto paper. Tony waits patiently, as an art therapist and understanding man, he knows I'll talk when I feel ready.

Through Autumn and into the early part of Winter, I attend groups at the centre, and work part-time. I especially look forward to the art therapy groups. Within the art sessions I find release and comfort, drawing my inner feelings and talking with Tony. During this time I'm also fighting even harder not to give in and self-injure.

Keep on fighting

It's important to recognise and praise every effort and success when trying to find alternatives to self-injury. Maybe you put off the act of injury for a few hours, maybe you did a deal and injured less than usual. If you have a set-back where you self–injure, be kind to yourself, as you would a friend. Ask yourself what you need. Maybe it is to phone a friend, to have a hot bubble bath or play music. It's important most of all to learn to care for yourself. If we don't love and respect ourselves how can we love and respect others?

One morning I arrive at the centre early, desperate to talk to Tony, or my doctor. I bang on the office door. A tall stranger opens the door.

'Hello, I'm Pete, the new staff nurse.'

'I wanted to...to.'

'Can I help?'

'No, I'm looking for Tony.'

'Tony's away on a course this week, would you like to talk with someone else?' I shrug, light a cigarette, trying to keep an air of calm.

'Can I talk to you then?'

I sit in the office opposite Pete.

'Would you like to tell me what's been happening then Jo?'

'I took my dad to the remembrance service this weekend, we watched the band. Dad said he wished I'd been a boy, and then I could have been in the Guards. I'm not good enough. Why can't he care for and protect me like when I was little? Why doesn't someone stand with me?'

'The person you need most is yourself. Keep positive Jo.'

'I'm sick of being strong. You don't understand.'

'In time maybe you'll let me understand you?' Pete replies.

'So how do I get through my work day tomorrow?'

'Imagine a parrot sitting on your shoulder, as your positive friend telling you you'll be okay.'

I think on these words a lot over the next few days.

'My parrot got sick!' I tell Pete the next time we meet at the centre. My arms are once again tightly bandaged.

Over the following weeks Pete keeps reassuring me, 'your self-injury doesn't make any difference to me. I'll still see you, talk to you, no matter what.' I'm shocked by Pete's words, more still by his calm acceptance of me. Unsure if this is too good to be true, I keep challenging Pete.

'So it doesn't matter how much I hurt myself?' I stand. 'You don't care.'

'Jo, sit down. I do care. Your safety is important, but I also respect your right to self-injure.'

I sit again, refuse to make eye contact with Pete.

'Would you like to talk about your friend self-injury?'

'My friend is my enemy. I've been up all night. The duty doctor talked about surgery, I was so scared. I rock my body, cradling my arm.

'Jo, I'm working with you, to enable you to make choices. One day self-injury will become a choice. In time you will be able to choose another way to communicate.'

I meet Pete's eyes for a moment.

Weeks pass, slowly I'm building trust, and starting to break the secrecy that surrounds my self-injury. Both with words and his patience and calm acceptance, Pete builds trust with me.

'I'm starting a little book of hope.' I tell Pete, 'I'm sick of destroying my body and surviving from one crisis to another.' The acceptance and unconditional care and respect I have from Pete are helping me increase the length of time between episodes of self-injury. As well as my little book, I'm working on artwork at home and at the centre.

'Your art work seems brighter.' Tony remarks to me.

'I'm learning to draw in an escape route or hope, even if I don't believe it.' My drawings are often still fragmented, dark, like my thoughts, but now there is a spark of life and hope in most of my sketches.

<u>Unconditional love</u>

Pete helped me with his direct, open approach. Most important was his unconditional respect and care for me. If you have a supporter or key worker, maybe you can negotiate safe boundaries and find out how they feel about self-injury. Communication is all-important.

It is also important to care for yourself in practical ways. Taking time out to relax, exercise and eat healthily. Keep trying to write, draw and develop safe ways to express your feelings.

Only a few weeks left to Christmas, I'm still fighting to keep clear of self-injury, with support from the art groups and talking to Pete. I join the other villagers struggling home against the first Winter gales.

Once home things are no easier, Mum phones with the news that my Uncle, Dad's brother, has died. Following the funeral David has more bad news for me.

'I've left my job.'

'Why? You've seemed settled there, it can't be that bad.'

David shrugs, late evening we huddle together on the settee.

That night, voices follow me, turning sleep into nightmares. The next day, determined to stop the voices screaming in my head, I clean the house.

'I can't sit anywhere.' David said, 'I'll get hoovered away.'

I'm unaware of time or place; know only that I must keep going to block out the screaming that fills me inside.

'Let's have a drink tonight.' I pour David a large home measure of Vodka and a double size for myself.

'Cheers, here's to us, survivors.'

The weekend passes in a haze of alcohol. Too many memories crowd my mind, too much pain to bear.

Monday morning I pass workmen putting up the Christmas tree in the village square. Bright coloured lights, tinsel sparkle against dark skies. I stand alone, unaware of early morning shoppers. My secret friend still beckons from the shadows.

- Acceptance - each person is unique, special in his or her own way. Each individual is worthy of care and attention. You do not need to work or justify your life to be special. You are alive, you are a miracle.
- It is important to keep going, to keep a perspective. There is no failure, only learning experiences. Each time we fall, we get up again and have learned from our mistakes.

- Try to keep a sense of humour, to keep a balance of activities. Plan into each day time for something fun and relaxing.
- Try to extend the time between the thoughts or urges to self-injure and the act of injury. STOP, name the feeling, own your feelings e.g. 'I feel angry.' Know that the feeling will pass. Remember every time you refrain from self-injury, or even injure less, is a victory. Keep fighting.

Chapter Six

Soft Light of Rainbows...Lessens my Pain

This New Year, I'm certain of the year's resolution.

'No more self-injury! I want to get my scars removed.' I announce to David.

'I hope you manage, your scars do look bad.' Filled with hope and determination, I also decide to leave the centre.

My doctor however has concerns, 'you sure you're okay Jo?'

'Yes I'm certain.'

'This is a major decision. Have you thought it through?'

'I'm sure. I'll be fine.' My resolve is unwavering. My doctor refers me to another doctor to have three minor operations to reduce scarring and pain. The first two operations go smoothly for me, apart from endless questions from concerned friends.

'Not again Jo?'

'Why have you cut again?'

The third operation is on the tenderest areas. My arm feels like it's on fire, the pain burns so deep.

'It will be worth it in the end,' David reassures me.

Later that night I lie awake, listening to David snoring. I think of Gran. Try to escape the pain in happier memories. I'm thinking of one of Gran's quotes as I finally drift to sleep. 'God tempers the wind to a shorn lamb, even though a naughty one.'

As soon as my arms have healed I'm back at work and planning coffee mornings to promote the self-help group. My mother Verity, work colleagues Angela and Sadie are regular supporters. Due to the small number of people attending the coffee mornings I decide to hold another open evening. 'We'll reach more people that way.' I'm intent on helping others like myself, who live the life of pain and shame that is self-injury.

Secrets

We have already looked at how the secret life of self-injury is damaging and hurtful. Try to trust one person, maybe your key nurse or doctor. Talk about your feelings prior to, during and after episodes of self-injury. Yes, this is scary to do but it is only through breaking the secrecy that we begin to heal. I know I'm not the only one. I know from the phone calls to the group line. After weeks of thinking of the best way to help, I decide I need to do more research into self-injury. I spend hours with cold coffee and a dictionary, reading books and articles in medical journals. I also subscribe to a magazine for people with self-injury difficulties.

In the second magazine received, an appeal by Jane – a Wiltshire based counsellor – grabbed my attention. She was seeking current and former self-harmers to participate in a research study for a book she was writing. The aim of the book was to examine why people turn to self-harm, and to explore helpful strategies for recovery. Throughout the winter months I wrote lengthy letters to Jane and, although we had never met, my trust in her gradually started to build. Verbalising distressing feelings is difficult for me, whereas writing is a useful safety valve – a way of letting out pain safely – art can work similarly too. While preoccupied with my letter writing or reading, David watches late night films.

'You'll be writing that book for Jane! Take a break, we'll go out for a drink.'

'Later, I'll finish this bit first.' Glancing up I notice David is drowning his loneliness in another home measure of Vodka.

As the weeks fly by, I pour out my heart in long letters to Jane, relating as much as I can remember of my life story. There are still memory gaps and partial memories that awaken me with painful nightmares. The gulf with David widens – emptiness from lack of communication.

Talk to me...

How often do those closest to us suffer when we stop talking? At this time I was too involved with the group and research to notice my husband's loneliness. At times I felt lonely too, so many feelings and thoughts inside. Try to keep talking to loved ones, friends, work colleagues, communication really does help. Talking helps us maintain and strengthen relationships. I know that when I've shut out others and tried to survive on my own the despair and desolation I felt threatened to overwhelm me. By having someone to share hopes and fears with we begin to feel more loved and secure.

First rays of Spring break dull days of Winter. David is busy planting seed in our back garden, today I join him. Aware of a coldness that separates us, I'm making an effort to help.

'Much help you are! That's my best rose, not weeds you've dug up. Go and make a pot of tea.'

Weeks pass, I throw myself into work and into organising the open evening to promote the group. I decide to write to invite Jane to give a talk based on her book. In the week leading up to the meeting I'm building my hopes, Jane's accepted my invitation. I'm also running from my fear of failure.

'I'll be late home tonight, overtime at work.'

'I'll turn out the spare room tomorrow evening.'

'Jo, stop! You look exhausted.' David tries in vain to halt my frantic activities.

If I could find words, I'd explain that I feel trapped by voices and painful memories, screaming inside my head. My moods fluctuate between feeling 'high' from living on the edge, and setting myself unrealistically high standards, to lows that motivate the need to self-injure. It feels almost as if I am caught on a roller coaster ride of pain, excitement, guilt and shame that is whirling out of my control.

<u>Are you riding an emotional roller coaster?</u>

Do you tend to be a perfectionist? Have difficulty in stopping work? Have to complete every single task before you can even consider taking a break? Take on impossible amounts of work or commitments? Pushing ourselves to the limits of our physical and emotional capabilities may be okay short term. For me it's often followed by self-injury. I fail to live up to my own ideals of perfection so I reject myself through self-injury.

The day of the open evening arrives. The village hall is nearly full as Jane starts her talk. I'm battling with voices screaming in my head to hear Jane's words. In a clear calm manner, Jane explains that people use self-injury as a survival strategy and how, contrary to popular belief, it serves as a suicide deterrent, and albeit temporarily, helps people feel better. She goes on to explain the role of dissociation in the process of self-injury, which her research findings suggested was a fairly common occurrence among those who engage in the act. She described dissociation as a skill developed by young children to cope with traumatic experiences. How in essence, they use it to 'mentally escape' from the reality of the situation, and the painful emotions associated with it. She continues that while dissociation serves as an extremely useful tool in childhood, it can cause problems in adulthood in that it becomes an automatic response to painful or stressful situations. In other words, a person may become overwhelmed with emotions and feel as if they are about to disintegrate, so they literally shut down emotionally (dissociate from the terrifying feelings or fear of disintegration). This can have the effect of making the person feel 'numb' (void of feelings) which is the desired effect. However, sometimes the feeling of numbness is so great that the person begins to doubt their existence or feels 'unreal', a very frightening feeling to experience. Thus self-injury is a way of confirming that they do exist, that they can bleed so they must be alive.

The next day after lunch, David and me see Jane back to the train station.

'I wish you could stay.' I hug Jane goodbye.

Inspired by Jane's talk, I spend time with my mother, talking about my childhood.

'I tried to be good, to help you Mum. I only wanted you to be happy again.'

'You were a good girl really Jo. I did what I did because I loved you. Gran tried to care for you, but she was elderly and frail, that's why you had to go into care for a time. Over the warm days of Summer we talk a little more. Talking and crying together is healing our past, even though it's painful.

Time

It is important to keep a balance of rest, relaxation and working. There is a danger of over enthusiasm leading to over work and exhaustion. When feeling physically burned out it is much harder to cope with any emotional issues. This was my pattern of 'Highs' then crash into self-injury. Learning to live more on a level, rather than a pattern of highs and lows takes time. Think of enjoyable activities, things you find relaxing and try to do at least one every day. Sleep is important, are you getting enough quality sleep regularly? Try to relax, unwind before going to bed. Establish a quiet, calm space in your evening to promote a good nights sleep.

I have mixed feelings at work too. I find solace in working and enjoy my friends Angela and Sadie's company. It's my confused feelings for Sadie that are hard for me to cope with. At times I wish Sadie could be farther away, other times I long for her to sit next to me. I remember my feelings for Maddy, the special close friendship we shared. How I longed for more as we reached our teenage years.

To manage these feelings of pain, fear unspoken love, I once again turn to my old friend self-injury. I fight the urge to cut for weeks, then a setback, with three visits to A&E within one month.

I'm running, screaming, crying, the pain is deep, shame is dark. Tears run, splashing in the rain. Blade flashes, pain then peace. Peace doesn't last; pain comes again.

'I'm sorry, I know I let you down again.' I say these words again and again over the next few weeks as friends and family hug and shout at me.

'Why?'

'What did we do to deserve this?'

'You let us down.'

David though is determined to stay with me, no matter what.

'I'll always be here. You need to think Jo, you'll lose your job. Maybe even lose use of your arms.' David hugs me after yet another trip to A&E.

The following morning at work, Sadie is waiting for me.

'You've a meeting with the boss at nine o'clock, good luck.'

'You're one of our best workers, but we can't go on like this. We never know if you'll be in or fit to work Jo. It's the end of the line. We thought you'd learned to control your self-harming.'

'I'm sorry. It's something I can't stop. I can't explain why.' I fight back tears as the manager tells me to collect my cards on the way out.

The next week I have an appointment to see my doctor.

'I noticed it was after I'd been on holiday that you cancelled your appointment. I've not seen you since. Were you angry with me for going away Jo?'

'I wanted you to stay. To care enough to be there for me. I did feel angry.'

'Will you keep your appointments and sort things out this time Jo? I also understand you've lost your job through taking time off due to self-injury. I think it's time you started to be honest with me so I can help you.'

On my next visit I start to explain.

'My mother was ill. I built an imaginary world and dreams to survive the pain and uncertainty.'

'What were your dreams Jo?'

'I wanted my Dad to take me away, away from mother's tears, and words I couldn't understand. Sometimes I think of you in that way. I was angry too, that you'd left me alone. I was scared that if I told you, you would turn me away, so I didn't come back... not 'till now.'

'Do you have plans Jo?'

'No, I survive one day to the next.'

'What about returning to the centre?'

After a couple of weeks of hunting I find temporary work at a warehouse on the outskirts of the village. It's hot, heavy work in cramped conditions. One morning as the temperature soars, I strip off my jumper, hoping the others are too busy to notice my arms.

'What happened?'

'I used to tame tigers,' I shout back. The supervisor pales, walks quickly away. Thankfully she leaves me alone, no further questions.

With encouragement from my doctor, I attend one day a week at the centre. Once more, Tony's art therapy group provides a safe place for me to explore difficult feelings. In the art therapy group I feel accepted, understood, listened to and believed. The other clients are supportive and show empathy to me. As everything discussed is confidential I'm able to build trust and learn to relate to others experiences. I also find Pete, the staff nurse I used to talk to accepting and patient.

'I feel safe here. You seem to understand a lot.' I confide in Pete. 'I don't know if I'll ever be free form self-injury.'

'You're learning all the time Jo. Every time you beat that urge to cut you're making progress,' Pete said.

'I'm fighting a loosing battle. Every time I cut I fail. I'm useless.'

'I'll still be here for you, whether you self-injure or not. I respect you unconditionally.

I start to share some of my poems and drawings with Pete. Also for the first time I share my thoughts of cutting.

'I have concerns for your safety. I feel for you when you hurt so deeply, but I'll always listen.' Pete reassures me again and again.

'Will you listen to the crazy stuff?' I ask. Pete nods as he leans towards me.

'When I cut it's as if I'm in another world. It's a place where time stands still. In the silence I slice through layers of guilt, anger, pain, shame to exquisite relief. From these broken pieces I emerge whole. My body is broken, yet my inner child has been both punished and soothed. Only now do I feel able to face the world. Cutting is my way of coping, but at a terrible cost, both physically and emotionally.

I muddle through the last days of Summer.

'I can't stand that warehouse much longer.' I tell David.

'You need to stick at it until you find something better. We can't afford for you to be off work too long. Remember your doctor's bills.' I chase after work, like I chase after hope. Hope for me is a dream that always ends too soon. Always out of reach.

A dream of peace, that seems unreal, like a rainbow in the mists of pain and shame.

- Healing by words, not wounds - every time you stop yourself from self-injury, even for a few minutes is a success. In time you will find you are able to make choices. Self-injury will change from being an automatic response to emotional pain to choice, to unhealthy choice.
- When you are troubled by difficult or painful memories or flashbacks, remember to hold onto reality. Put your feet firmly on the ground, tell yourself 'I am an adult now. Things are different. I can choose to care for myself.'
- Remember to keep a balance, to plan rest and relaxation into your daily routine.
- Trust - to build trust with those who are trying to support you takes time. Start by being honest. Check out how the other person thinks or feels about your self-harm. If they are really uncomfortable it may be possible to change your care worker.
- Try to lengthen the gap between the thought and urge to self-injure and the act of injury by asking yourself what you need. You may want to self-injure, but you may need space to talk, cry and express feelings in writing or art. You may need to phone a friend or get or give a hug. This gap between the thought and urge to self-injure may start at a very short time, maybe minutes. The longer the gap achieved, the more chance to see self-injury as a choice; that we have other choices, more positive ways of expressing feelings.

Chapter Seven

Hide in Shadows of Pain or Seek Rainbows of Hope?

Golden sun dances, warming our aching hearts. David and me shuffle through first fall of Autumn leaves, on our favourite woodland walk.

'I used to come here to dream' I hug David. 'I had dreams to be a nurse. I'd find cures for illness, so no-one need be in pain anymore.'

'It's never too late. You can change work. You keep saying you're fed up at that warehouse.' As we wander home David continues to encourage me.

Over the following weeks I apply to hospitals, care homes, schools. I tear another rejection letter up. That evening a small advert in the local paper catches my eye. 'Wanted, caring person to assist individuals with disabilities in family home environment.' Two weeks later I'm so excited as I get ready for my first day.

On my first day off, I visit my key nurse Pete to tell him my good news.

'I've started a new job as a care assistant.'

'That's great Jo, you're really doing well. You've been clear of self-injury for a long time too.'

'Things have never been so good and I love my work.'

'When the thoughts come back, what will you do?'

'They won't! I'll be okay.' I snap angrily.

'It's important to have choices, alternatives. Do you really believe you're totally free? That you'll never think of self-injury again Jo?'

'You always turn my thoughts upside down. I'm all right.'

'Think on choices Jo, I'll be here when you're ready to talk again.' Pete calmly folds his notes, never shows if I test his patience to the limit.

The first weeks at the home I often return home covered in paint, flour or ground.

'You having fun Jo?' David laughs with me as I shake glitter from my jumper.

'It's the best work ever. The folks up at the home always see the fun side of life. They ignore pain, wheelchairs, limitations they're great to be with.

'It's good to see you happy and relaxed.'

'I've found my place, I feel like I really belong at the home.'

Time at the home becomes increasingly special for me. More and more I think of the residents as my extended family. The sweet old gentleman is like a grandfather, the younger residents are my brothers and sisters. I care for them all with loving care, often doing extra bits of shopping or running errands in my own time.

'How's work going?' Pete asks the next time I call into the centre.

'It's really good, I think of the residents as the big family I always wanted. I used to feel lonely, being an only child.'

'Do you take your work home with you Jo? Do you have time for yourself?'

'I do posters, shopping, run errands in my own time. I don't need time for me.'

'You look tired Jo.'

'Don't criticise. I'm okay.' I curl up in my chair. Inside I feel shame at snapping back at Pete.

'Jo?'

'I don't want to talk.'

'Jo, you know I'm here. I'll listen when you're ready. You're doing well, but I'm sure there's something bothering you. Remember to phone if you need to talk.'

'I'm fine.' I shout as I run out.

Halfway home I slow to a walking pace, stare up at grey skies. Pete is the first person I've trusted, felt safe with for a long time. He's the only one who lets me talk whether I've cut or not. Maybe I told him too much? Does Pete understand too much? Self-injury was my secret life, my thoughts race.

'I'll be all right I tell myself.'

Inner secrets

We all have inner thoughts, dreams; it is important to find ways to express our inner feelings. My work at the home was

70

important to me in that I was fulfilling my childhood dreams of helping my mother when she was sad. Whenever one of the residents at the home was distressed or ill, I'd take extra special care of them. In doing so I was trying to help my memories of my mother being ill heal.

Late Autumn rushes past in a whirl of work and fallen leaves, first cold Winter winds come too soon. We take advantage of a break in the weather and my long weekend off to visit David's friend Simon.

Our weekend away passes in gales of laughter as David and Simon take the longest glider flight of the day, which we celebrate in Simon's local pub. Sunday afternoon we enjoy cream teas at the village teashop.

All too soon the weekend is over, David and me return to work. Following my first day at work, I stumble in through the door.

'What a shift! I've not stopped all day. You all right David?'

David stares out of the window, unusually silent.

'I've lost my job. So much for my plans to get the supervisor's post.'

'I'm sorry.' I reply. Inside I'm scared, screaming. Will David get ill again? I know that David feels insecure at times, that the routine of work is important to him. Through the following weeks we lead neat, tidy lives, the house and garden are tidy and clean, yet our home is filled with an uneasy silence.

'It's Christmas in two weeks, let's have both families round here.'

'We could.' David agrees reluctantly.

Christmas day, with our big family gathering and David seems to have forgotten his troubles.

'A real traditional Christmas, this is kind of you both.' David's mother hugs us.

'Come on Jo, we'll do these.' Verity, my mother clatters piles of dishes into our kitchen.

'It's just like Christmas at Gran's, Dad always had a sleep and we'd do the washing up.'

'You still miss your Gran don't you Jo?' Mother hugs me.

'Every day.'

'I do too, she was really special.'

Life, love and tears

When Gran died my search for love, acceptance and hope
began. I craved affection, blamed myself for Gran's death. I
began to hate my life. I hated my body for being alive when Gran
was dead.

Inside of me, my inner child cries, I can't find words to express
the pain and shame I feel.

When I allow myself tears, I wash my pain away, feel relief.

When I paint small delicate flowers I find peace in remembering
Gran's garden. I'm trying to remember and celebrate the happy
memories in order to let go of the pain I feel.

New year sweeps in with a light dusting of snow. The second
January Sadie phones.

'Hi Jo, how's tricks? It's Angela's birthday Saturday. Will you
and David meet us? We're having a surprise party.'

'Yes okay, eight o'clock did you say?'

On the day of the party David decides to stay at home. The
lounge bar of the local pub is transformed with streamers,
banners and balloons.

'You didn't have to go to all this trouble.' Angela giggles.

'You're only twenty one once.'

Laughing, dancing, joking with my old friends, I feel relaxed
and happy. In the smokey atmosphere of the pub, I try to talk to
Sadie.

'Sadie?'

'Shout Jo, I can't hear, the music's too loud.'

'Nothing.' I reply. I watch longingly as Sadie's golden hair
sparkles in the disco lights. I shouldn't feel this way about Sadie,
I tell myself as I walk home. With David still out of work, it's
another excuse to take on extra hours at work. I'm also the first
to volunteer for extras like helping out at fetes, cake sales or
outings.

'Do you sleep Jo?'

'How do you find time to do all this?'

Other staff start to show concern at my lengthy hours. If I could
have found words maybe I'd have shared my secret thoughts.

Voices screaming in my head, guilty, you're wrong to crave love. If I could take away your pain, could I wash away my shame? If I could wipe away your tears, could I banish my fears? Is this your pain or mine? Long, lonely nights these thoughts keep me awake. I'm judge, jury and executioner to myself. I find myself guilty of not loving my mother enough. If I'd been a good girl, if I'd told someone, would Gran have died that night? If I could find words, the right words? From daybreak, to evening I never stop. While at work, nursing the residents I often see pain in their eyes... my pain or your pain?

'Jo, you've been down like this before. Go and see your nurse, Pete isn't it? David first asks, and then demands me to seek help.

'I'm doing fine. Leave me alone.'

I'm lost in a vicious circle of guilt, pain and despair. Memories crowd my mind.

'Be a good girl, listen to mummy.'

I listened for seventeen years until our pain blurred.

Drawing boundaries

A big part of my self-injury has been about drawing boundaries, between others and myself. Following abuse of any kind it is common for individuals to feel soiled, used and that a part of them has been taken away. Although self-injury may be helping you survive unbearable feelings of loss, anger and shame, please consider other ways of drawing boundaries. If you have been abused, first seek professional counselling. Art, music or writing may also help as safe outlets for difficult feelings.

February gales blow the last wisps of snow. David and me are together, yet apart. We're both spiralling down into a mist of depression. Desperate to share my fears with someone, I visit my key nurse Pete at the centre.

'I've been thinking about cutting again, I'm scared.'

'What's been happening Jo?'

'Not much, I've been busy at work. I'll be okay.'

'There's more to this than a busy shift at work isn't there?' Pete asks.

'I'm sorry. I can't explain, I thought I'd be able to.'

'Think on alternatives Jo, try writing your thoughts on paper if you're not ready to talk. Don't even bother about spelling or grammar, just write what's in your head. Remember I'll be here when you're ready to talk.'

'I'm going out for a walk. Need to clear this headache.' I tell David later that evening. The church clock strikes eleven as I stagger round the church square. My legs burn, my arms feel wet and sticky. Moonlight flickers, casting light into dark corners.

Into this empty space, voices scream, echoing form empty shops.

'Jo, it's David, come home with me.' I hear words through a deep fog of dissociation. I make no response, carry on walking.

'Jo.' David shouts, 'Come over here.'

'I need help.' I hold out my arms.

The now familiar trip to A&E department follows. I know the routine.

'Why this time?'

'Don't cry.'

Still in a state of dissociation, reality far away, I cry. Unable to talk, I rest my head on David's shoulder.

Don't cry,

When life seems unreal, you call to me.

Shadows haunt, head spins, light breaks.

'Come to me, run to me, I'll set you free.'

My secret friend lets my pain out.

Blood cleanses, wounds scream. Do you see?

A child in pain. My shame? You shout...

Don't cry.

My memories mingle with the doctor's words.

'Bad girls cry, bad children go to hell.' I learn not to cry. I touch my scars, each one of them tells a story, each one a piece of jigsaw, a note of pain. I promised, I swore, yet I've cut again.

When the blackness descended like a total eclipse, when it seemed there was no-one around I hid. I cut. You found me.

Somehow despite my protests you cleaned my wounds. You believed in me, kept believing in me. Please don't give up, there is a tiny flicker of hope that keeps flickering in the darkness. We need to hold onto this hope however fragile. Each person has a purpose, a meaning, their own unique journey to make. No-one else can take your place. My cycle of self-injury spins tighter, more frequent, and more severe.

The next day I'm back at work.

'It's a slip. It won't ever happen again. I don't need time off sick.' I try desperately to convince my boss to save my job.

'You need to look at ways of coping, Jo. We need to know you're reliable. As you're a good worker, I'll let this incident pass with a warning.'

'How did work go?' David asks me later.

'Okay, I've still got my job.'

'I've got good news too. I start a new job Monday next week.'

Through the last days of Winter, David settles into his new work. I'm working harder than ever, determined to prove my worth. Evenings find us slumped on the settee, both exhausted.

Sunday is David's gardening day. 'Look Jo, we've got the first Daffodils coming in that sheltered spot.'

'Can I take some?' I pick a handful of Daffodils and snowdrops and wander slowly to the village churchyard.

Neatly trimmed grass now covers Gran's grave. I lay my bunch of flowers.

'I'm sorry it's taken so long. I couldn't come before.' I touch the cold headstone, finding no comfort or reassurance there I kneel on damp grass for a few minutes. A cool breeze blows my fears away.

'I brought you our first daffodils Gran.' My step is lighter on the way home. I've found that saying goodbye is a step towards healing.

Back at work, the residents are looking forward to Spring. This year a special Easter parade is planned, the whole village community is encouraged to take part.

'We need a volunteer to organise the home's entry and participation.'

'I'll do it.' I leap in impulsively. Four other staff also volunteer to help.

'This is the first Easter parade for ten years. The home must be well represented. Can you manage Jo?'

'Yes, we'll be stars. We'll have costumes, music and transport organised well ahead of time.'

'Don't forget to ask about wheelchair access Jo.'

'I'll phone the main organiser this evening.' I reassure my boss, determined to prove I've made a fresh start. Inside I have doubts, will my past shadow my efforts or can I continue to seek rainbows of hope?

Summary

- To identify that the screaming inside my head is from my inner child was a big step forward for me. To understand that is where my strongest feelings originate, that my trapped emotions of anger, guilt and pain are from years of pent up feelings.
- We need to accept our feelings, they are not good or bad. Feelings are indicators of what needs addressing in our lives. When we try to push feelings away or bury them, they grow stronger and more intense.
- To talk about our deepest feelings may seem too scary, especially at first. Maybe you could try sharing your artwork or writing with someone you trust.

Chapter Eight

Broken Inside, Desperately Clutching at Rainbows of Hope

Frantic activity fills the week before the Easter parade. I laugh off feelings of frustration and panic.

'So what if only one other person has a costume ready.'

'Jo, you've got two days and fifteen outfits to get ready!'

I count residents and costumes, remembering my counting game from years ago. I was a teenager, rocking silently, counting relatives, pleading, bargaining with God not to take another. Six deaths within two years. I decide to shop at the charity shops, it's too late now to hand-sew costumes. Friday afternoon I hand out the last costume.

'It's still not enough. You're still bad.' Voices scream in my head. I run home to David.

'It's almost Easter and I haven't spring cleaned yet!' I shout, grabbing a bucket and cloths.

'No need to make work Jo, the house looks okay. I'm painting at the weekend if you want something to do.'

Saturday finds me wobbling on a ladder as I stretch out to paint the garage wall.

'Careful Jo, you're splashing paint on my Dahlias.'

'Where?' I playfully splash paint on David's boots.

Sunday evening, having painted, cleaned and tidied house and garden David is relaxing with a mug of cocoa. I'm still restless.

'You'll wear a hole in that carpet! Settle down Jo.'

'I'm scared. Will tomorrow be okay?'

'You'll be fine Jo, the parade is only a bit of fun.'

Throughout the long night I count costumes, residents, volunteers. Panic fills my mind, have I done enough? Once more I find I'm pushing myself to perfection. I order to keep my job I've taken on extra hours and responsibility for organising the parade. All I want is to feel accepted. I'm desperate for someone to say 'I care. I accept you.' Maybe if I'd shared my fears with David? Maybe if I'd asked for support from my friends at work? Maybe if I could share my fears I could sleep.

Keeping a balance

Do you find yourself taking on impossible amounts of work?
Extra responsibility? Are you crying out for love and acceptance
from others, but too ashamed to admit it? We all need affection
and love, it's part of being human. We can start by taking care of
ourselves. When we begin to treat ourselves with respect others
will follow. Try to rebuild your self-esteem. Each day remind
yourself 'I am a worthwhile person. I am valuable. I am unique
and special.

Easter Monday morning, even the light drizzle can't dampen
the enthusiasm of the crowd already gathering.
'Over here,' the marshal waves the home's minibus in. Trudy,
the home's youngest resident is first out. Two o'clock, the sun
has burnt off the mist, leaving clear blue skies and packed
streets.
'We're at the front Jo, hurry up.' Trudy shouts to me. The
village band strikes up a merry tune. Cheerleaders follow,
batons twirling, proud parents waving.
'It's our turn.' Trudy and me lead the home's entry, sailors and
soldiers. As the parade marches along cobbled streets, crowds
scatter flowers. Mrs Smith, the sweet shop owner throws sweets
to the children.
'Jo, Jo! Over here.' I catch a glimpse of my parents, Verity and
Jeff, waving and cheering at the back of the crowd. By the end
of the afternoon we are exhausted. Trudy holds the silver cup
high.
Later that evening I meet David in the village tearooms. 'Good
day Jo?'
'Great, we won first prize.'
'There's Sadie and Angela.'
After a few minutes chatting David decides to leave.
'Come on Jo, let's go and get a drink to celebrate your
success.' I eagerly follow Sadie and Angela to the pub.
'Here's to us.'
'Best mates forever.'
After several more rounds I stand to toast the crowded bar.
'You're all my best mates.'

Celebration of life

The residents at the home taught me to celebrate life, to appreciate every day. Through their courage and sense of humour, no matter how much pain they were in, to live each day to the full. It is so easy to get discouraged when we fail, when our hopes are dashed, there is no failure only learning experiences. The only failure is in not getting back up again. We cannot change our past, yesterday is gone and tomorrow is yet to come. By living in the present moment we can reduce tension and begin to celebrate life.

Nine o'clock the next morning church bells clang. 'I'm dead, this must be hell.' Through glazed eyes I see David. 'What are you doing here?'
'Trying to sleep if you'll get the phone.'
'Jo, it's Mum, your Dad's poorly, can you come around?' My mother's anxious voice pierces the muzzy haze in my head. Later that morning I'm recovering with mugs of strong coffee.
'You look worse than I did first thing.' My Dad laughs with me.
'I was celebrating the home winning first prize. You feeling better then Dad?'
'I'm fine, just been doing a bit too much. I've nearly finished painting the outside walls.'
'I'll help you Dad. I'm a dab hand at painting.'
I jot a note to phone Dad on my next day off. My offer to help is soon forgotten though as I take on overtime at work. A week later I remember and phone my parents.
'Mum, it's Jo, I'll be round tomorrow to help dad with the painting.'
'Don't bother. Your Dad's finished. He's exhausted. It's been too much for him to do it all on his own.'
I slam the phone down. Bang my head against the wall. I feel so much pain and rejection.
I'm feeling rejected by David too, he has an offer for a two weeks training course in London.
'If all goes well, I'll get promoted, then there could be further courses.'

'That's great.' I hide my feelings well, years of practice. David is happy, I can't spoil that by sharing my fears.

'Extra shift Jo?'

'Can you get shopping, collect these prescriptions?' At least I'm appreciated at work I tell myself.

Communication

Due to a lack of communication between myself and David, and my parents, our lives are becoming increasingly difficult. It's important to check out what the other person is thinking or feeling, not just to assume the worst. Often it takes courage to ask a partner or friend for their opinion. From experience though it's proved valuable, as I've received far more support and care than the rejection I feared.

As the May Day bank holiday approaches I'm torn between work and getting the group stand ready for the May Day fair.

May Day holiday and the village green is filled with families, laughing, chatting happily. The village fair is in full swing as I set up the group stand at the edge of the charity area. The other stalls are busy, yet when people read 'Self-Harm Self-Help Group' they turn quickly away.

'You're even less cuddly than protect the hedgehogs!' My friend Angela laughs with me.

Later that afternoon, my thoughts turn to running and self-injury. I have unspoken fears of David leaving me, my fears of rejection from my parents and the long afternoon of rejections for my group stand. In late afternoon shadows I fall through layers of feelings... anger, pain, shame, guilt. My inner pain and fear of abandonment, a small child crying... 'Where's mummy?'

In an effort to stop these thoughts, I continue my frenzied activity over the next few weeks. The voices are back, screaming inside my head.

'Before you die, you must be clean. Let blood wash out evil.'

I have an explosion of sounds that terrorise me by day and blur into haunting nightmares.

On my next day off I visit Pete, my key nurse at the day centre.

'Hi Jo, not seen you for ages, how are you?' Pete's words join the orchestra of noise in my head, fighting for attention. Lost in desperation I shake my head.

'I don't feel right. I'm scared.'

'Why are you scared Jo?'

'I'm scared of my anger. My group stand at the May Day fair was a disaster! People want help, but they don't want to support the charity.' I grip my chair. Pete's quiet, calm manner usually calm me, today it's different.

'You know you can talk to me whether you self-injure or not?' I nod. Even now this idea is alien to me. For years both friends and family have used bribes and threats to try to stop my self-injury. Pete's acceptance is different.

Pete leans forward. 'I'm concerned for your safety Jo. Is your friend self-injury getting out of control?'

'Leave me alone. You don't know anything.'

'Are you hurting inside Jo? Does your anger hide pain?'

'You ask daft questions!' I shout, slamming the office door.

That evening I sit on the garden wall as darkness falls and I fall back into memories… I'm about nine years old, it's a bitterly cold Winters day and I'm sitting next to mother on a park bench. Sitting, listening, after a while my legs feel numb like they're not they're anymore. I wiggle my toes and make small movements to keep warm. I know if I keep mother talking to me we'll be okay. That in time she will get up and we'll go home. I learn to hold on, to believe in my strength, resilience and patience to keep going.

During the next week, I work overtime at work, clean the house and take group phone calls, all through a haze of pain. Friday afternoon I have a half-day, David is out at work.

'Come to me, run, hide, escape, cut, cleanse, die.' Voices scream inside my head hour after hour.

'You must die, cleanse first, I'll find you, kill you.'

'Give yourself completely.'

The voices continue as I buy my tools from the shop. I'm only dimly aware of the damp, cramped public toilet. My chosen place to escape. I fall into blackness, black stinking hell of survival. Silent screams resound against cold walls dripping with condensation and fear. Shattered dreams pierce ragged wounds. Pain thumps to the voices in my head. Falling into a gap between life and death. Somewhere between heaven and hell I find peace. Cleansed, my spirit flies free.

'Everything is beautiful.' Silence fills the empty space and the comforting blanket of dissociation protects me from reality. Into this half world, the evening cleaners clattering mops and buckets bring me closer to reality. Frantically I clean the cubicle, wrap my arms tightly, and hide my tools in my pockets. I slip into cool evening shadows. I have no memory of arriving at A&E or how I got there.

'Jo, what happened?' the nurses ask. I hear words, but they make no sense.

'We'd better phone her husband.'

Nurses bustle around and I'm vaguely aware of a doctor stitching my arms. David too seems like a stranger as he holds my hand as I'm transferred to the psychiatric hospital. Three or four days pass in a muddle of unasked and unanswered questions. Who am I? Where am I? Why?

<u>Broken inside</u>

At times when we are overwhelmed by emotions it can be difficult to know what we do feel. Pete, my nurse, was the only one to see through my aggressive and angry façade to see the broken child within. I was using my anger as a protective cage so that others could not see that inside I was crying, hurt and lonely. Even at this time when I feel broken inside, there is a spark that refuses to die. I believe that this spark is my inner child. I believe that we all have an inner child, that this cannot be destroyed by alcohol, self-injury or by being ignored. This inner child, this spark of love, beats inside no matter what. It's also the first time I realise the impact my self-injury has on my inner child.

In the darkness my child lies
In the stillness my child cries
When I cut...
My child dies.

One afternoon my parents visit, I fetch mugs of coffee for them.

'I'm sorry.' I wipe at the spilt drinks with my jumper sleeve. 'I didn't think you'd come.' I swallow hard against tears.

'Jo, it's all right. Of course we came. We still love you.'

During the second week of my stay in hospital I receive a letter from my boss at work.

'Sorry, but we feel unable to keep your job open.' The words leap off the page and thump in my head.

'I can't see my friends or the residents at work. I've lost my job.' I tell David between sobs.

'You'll soon get another job.'

'The folks I nursed were my family, I loved them. I wanted to make a difference.'

'Jo, it's okay.' David hugs me. I cry.

'I've let my residents down.' For days I can't eat, sleep or settle to rest. I can see no way forward. No hope.

One evening, one of the night staff shows me a new book on self-injury. 'SAFE, the breakthrough healing program for self-injurers.' The stories of recovery in the SAFE book are inspiring. To know that people in a worse state than me have gone on to make a full recovery is exciting.

Monday morning, I'm back at the day centre and eager to show Pete my new book. 'This time I want to break free, to make a new life without cutting.'

With support from the day centre, and encouragement from David, I'm working through the first part of the SAFE program. This consists of fifteen writing assignments that I find both challenging and exhausting e.g. SAFE assignment, the emotions surrounding self-injury:

Q1. What feelings and fantasies do I typically have prior to, during and after an episode of self injury?

Q2. What feelings have I wanted to create in others through this?

Q3. What feelings do I elicit from others even if I don't intend to?

I'm also finding writing a release of tension and pain, a way of expressing thoughts and feelings. Through the assignments, I'm making sense of memories and feelings. Seeing patterns and rituals to my self-injury are helping me grow and heal. The main focus of the SAFE program is on taking responsibility for your own life and actions. After years of blaming others, or some mysterious force for my self-injury, I find this idea difficult.

<u>Taking responsibility</u>

As a child I was not to blame for my mother's illness. It took me a long time to accept this. As adults, however, we are responsible for our choices in how we handle events. We can choose to see unpleasant events as learning experiences. We can make decisions and goals in order to make our lives better. Make a dream, hold onto your dream, work towards that dream. Let your dream hold you through the bad days we all have.

During one of the art therapy groups I also decide to share my secret feelings of love and longing for Sadie and, years before, for my friend Maddy. I paint a woman, clothed in pink ribbons standing in a mist of tears.
'What's your picture about?' Tony asks me.
'Forbidden love. I love my friend Sadie. I wish we could be more than just friends. I wish she would... but we never could.' I look at Tony. He sits next to me.
'I'm a terrible person. Evil.' I tell Tony, determined to reject and condemn myself first.
'Jo, you're entitled to your feelings.' Tony's calm acceptance surprises me, even though he was the one I chose to trust. As days pass I realise that in sharing my secret I've lessened the pain and guilt I feel inside.

Over the next weeks, I share some of my assignments with Pete.
'It's good to see you using words to express your feelings, rather than self-injury.'
'It's hard, especially at the moment. I've got PMT, but I bet you don't believe me'

84

'You could see June, a new nurse, she could help your PMT with aromatherapy.'

Two weeks later, I have my first appointment to see June. Her calm, patient manner eases my fears. Despite these changes, life at home with David is tense.

'Where are you going?'

'When will you be back?'

'I feel like you're my jailor!' I snap at David.

'I need to know.'

'You're forever checking up on me.' I thump the kitchen table in frustration.

'How can I trust you Jo? I'm scared. I live in constant fear for your safety.' I meet David's eyes and see torment and exhaustion.

'David, I'm sorry.'

'Every time you lied to me, trust died.'

'I've said I'm sorry.'

'You could be left permanently disabled or worse.'

'I wish I could promise you I'd never self-injure again. This time scared me too.'

The next day at the centre I share my fears of returning to self-injury and losing David with Pete.

'What can I do? I need to change. How can me and David live without trust?'

'Where is it cast in stone that you can never give up self-injury?' Pete looks straight at me as he challenges me. Although I've felt challenged by the SAFE program to take control of my life, Pete's direct approach hits me hard. The combination of realising the pain I've caused David, my family, and this challenge from Pete gives me a lot to think about.

I've reached a crossroads in my journey. I have choices, to complete the SAFE program to give up my identity as a self-injurer. I know it's a major decision to make, that to succeed I need to change my life completely.

Later that afternoon, David and me are out walking.

'Look over there, a rainbow. Quick. It's fading.' I turn to see David's rainbow, see tears in his eyes. I hug David. I'm running out of time to rebuild my life and stay with David.

Rainbows of hope are there, will you reach out?

Summary

• By identifying and reclaiming our inner child we find hope to break free from the cycle of self-injury. Healing begins with listening to our inner child, with love and acceptance. Whatever happened as a child we were unable to change, we can now take control as adults. As adults we can break this cycle of blame and abuse through acceptance and love.

• We will always have highs and lows to life, change is inevitable. It is important only to keep going, to believe that you do have a future. If you return to self-injury, remind yourself that it is only a setback and that you are worth more than a life of pain.

• We can manage self-injury by use of an advocate. Write positive thoughts about yourself and keep it in your purse or pocket. Read at times when you feel vulnerable to self-injure.

• Work on understanding self-injury more. Keep a note of triggers. When are you most at risk form self-injury? What time of day? Places? Are certain people involved? Thoughts, feelings, voices, stress? The more we understand and share about our self-injury the less power it has over our lives.

Chapter nine

Dancing on rainbows

Hot Midsummer's day, bright sunlight pierces the dull ache of pain I feel as I walk to the Centre. As I stroll I'm reflecting on my weekend with David. Anxious days filled with endless questions.

'Did you buy anything you shouldn't?'

'When will you be home?'

I have to change, try to rebuild trust, my thoughts whirl. The SAFE program has given me hope. I can change. Nearing the centre, I look up. In the distance, a rainbow stretches from land to sea. In that moment my decision is made.

'Pete, I need to ask for your help.' I perch on the office chair, fearing rejection.

'The last part of my SAFE program is a goodbye ritual to my life of self-injury. Would you come with me?'

'I feel honoured you asked me Jo. I take that as a compliment.'

Friday afternoon, I'm pacing the empty hall, waiting for Pete. The other clients have long gone, leaving me alone with my thoughts and fears.

'You ready then Jo?'

'Yes, I'll meet you at the headland.'

A light breeze blows through my hair as Pete and me scramble down the rocky headland to the beach.

'I'll wait here.' Pete sits quietly. I wander closer to the sea.

'Goodbye my friend.' I whisper as I throw pink rose petals into crashing waves.

'Goodbye Gran.' I break the last rose, stroking its soft petals, thorns scratch tender scars. I turn, Pete stands as if ready to leave.

'Roses Jo?'

'Gran loved roses. She had a huge rose bush in her front garden, beautiful white roses. When I was little I'd save the petals for my doll's wedding.' I turn to look out to sea. 'Pink roses were Gran's favourite though.'

Waves lap at my feet, Pete jumps back. Salt spray stings my face. For a moment I long to disappear.

'Cutting helped me survive, now I'm choosing to live. I've often come here to this headland, when I've felt lost or confused.'

'You chose the right place and way to say goodbye then.' Today as always Pete is calm and patient. 'We can talk about today next week if you like Jo.'

'See you Monday.' I choke back tears with a cough, it's been an emotional afternoon for me.

Choosing to live

My decision to say goodbye to my life of self-injury sets me free to re-build my life. Instead of focusing on hurting myself and blocking feelings, I'm making a fresh start. Once we make the decision to end self-injury we are free to learn to feel again. Having blocked feelings for years it's a challenge and an exciting journey to take.

Saturday morning I visit my parents.

'Hi Jo, how's things? Time for coffee?'

Over coffee I share my news.

'I've given up self-injury forever.'

'We hope you stay well Jo.'

Mother's voice trembles as she hugs me. David too seems unsure.

'I want to trust you, it's not easy. You've let me down so many times.' I hug David close.

Monday morning, I return to the centre eager to talk with Pete, to share my feelings about my goodbye ritual to self-injury.

'I've only got a few minutes today Jo. I've got to get my paperwork up to date for my holiday next week. How've you been over the weekend?'

'I felt angry when I said goodbye.'

'You didn't appear angry Jo.'

'I couldn't say. It felt like a funeral service, for the old me, the way I used to be.'

'A lot of change Jo.'

'I feel like I've lost my identity.'

'You're doing well Jo, keep calm. You'll be all right. Do you still talk to your mum?'

'I haven't lately, maybe it would help.'

'We'll talk more when I get back from my holidays in three weeks.'

Partly through the SAFE assignments, also talking to my mother, I'm now understanding and accepting my past. I know my mother loved and cared for me the best way she could.

'There was no-one to talk to.'

Mother weeps softly as she rocks in her chair. To see my mother distressed hurts me. Yet, breaking secrets and years of silence is bringing us closer together.

'I love you mum.' Three words I thought I'd never say and mean.

The decision to love

Daily we can decide to forgive ourselves and others who may have hurt us. In doing so we set ourselves free from the powerful grip of the past. Forgiveness, I have found, is a process rather than a one-time decision. By holding onto past hurts we chain ourselves to past painful memories. In letting go we can start each new day afresh. My decision to follow through the SAFE program and have a ritual goodbye ceremony to self-injury was a part of my letting go of my old life and starting anew.

It's a tribute to my mother Verity, my doctor and staff at the centre that we are able to talk again. For three months after I left home, I refused to visit or even talk to my mother. My years of self-injury have damaged relationships, not least between my parents and me. Through talking with my mother, I now understand some of the torment my parents suffered.

Friday morning in the art group at the day centre, I'm making a box.

'Unusual project for you Jo.' Tony watches as I carefully fold and glue card.

'I used to put all my bad feelings in a box, chain the box and throw away the key.'

'Bad feelings Jo?'

'My feelings of anger, hurt, sadness, insecurity. My feelings for Sadie and Maddy.'

'Why?'

'To survive, I had to shut out everything. In blocking out the bad stuff, I shut out love.'

Life, laughter and love

In blocking our feelings, through dissociation we lose touch with reality. I found that I lost the ability to feel love, to laugh, to cry during my years of self-injury. Try to reach out to others now that you are breaking free. In sharing we find happiness and peace. Simple pleasures like a cup of tea and a chat, phone a friend or visit an elderly neighbour.

The week is over, I look to Pete as he packs his briefcase, 'Have a good holiday.'

'I'll see you in three weeks Jo.' Pete pauses, 'You okay?'

'Just tired. I've had a lot of nightmares recently.'

'To dream good dreams, think of flying.' Pete said.

'Think of flying, dream of being free.' I whisper these words to myself as I fall exhausted to sleep that night.

Over the next two weeks I start to put poems and sketches together in a folder to show Pete on his return from holiday. It's a small step, yet important for me. I've many half-finished artworks and projects. To live for today and make plans for tomorrow is a new idea after years of self-injury. The main focus of the SAFE program now is on moving on, setting small goals to achieve.

David too is busy making plans. 'I've got funding for my two weeks training package. It's great. When I get back, I'll get promotion too.' David looks to me, clearly expecting praise and excitement.

'I love you. I'm happy for you.' I hug David and bury my head in his shoulder to hide my tears.

Hours later, listening to David snoring, I talk to my bear.

'I'll lose David. He won't need me. He has a wonderful new job. What can I offer? It'll all fall apart, like when mum found someone else.

I remember the jealousy I felt when my mother first found someone else to talk to. Though my role as child counsellor was unwanted it was the only way I knew to relate to my mother.

The following week is my first aromatherapy session with June. Soft music, healing oils and June's calm acceptance all help me feel at ease. At the end of the session June asks 'Can I rub oil on your scars Jo? It'll help them heal.' I pull my arms close to my chest. I stare at my arms. A mesh of red raised twisted scars.
'Only if you'd like.'
June cups a small dish of oil in her hands. I've never let anyone touch my arms, except out of desperate medical need. In learning to trust, I'm letting others close enough to heal my pain, both physical and emotional. Tears splash onto my shirt. My shoulders shake with years of pent up emotion. Curling up into a ball, I turn away. There is no time, only an empty space of pain and tears. After a while I cough, 'I'm sorry.'
'It's all right to cry. It's normal.' June rests her hand on my shoulder.
'I could only cry after I'd cut. Then at A&E the doctor would tell me off, he probably thought I was feeling sorry for myself. I didn't. After I cut was the only time I could cry, to let out my pain.'

<u>Time</u>
Time is precious, a gift.
You touch my scars, accept my pain.
I learn to trust, discard my shame.
Bitter tears I cry, regret and loss.
You touch my hand, there is no blame.
Your gentle touch heals my pain.
I learn to talk, feel whole again.
Many tears I cry, a woman's shame.
You touch my heart... I cry again.

During the week following my first aromatherapy, I continue to work on my art project. I remember as a child making books for Gran. Little books of pictures and poems, prepared with the enthusiasm and innocence of a child. I have happy memories, so proud to give Gran my best collections of pictures and poems.

Friday evening, I tie my art project together with yellow ribbons.

'You've done well there Jo. It's nice to see you taking an interest in art again.' David hugs me.

'I can't wait until Monday, to see Pete and show him too.'

Monday morning, I'm surprised when Tony calls me into the office.

'Pete's delayed back from holiday.' Tony shuffles, seems tense.

'He's coming back though? Pete is coming back?'

'I can't say for sure, at the moment we can only tell you he's delayed.'

I throw my art folder in my bag. Choking back tears I slam the office door.

Every day I attend the centre I steal a glance at the office. 'Surely today Pete will be back?' Days blend into weeks, my art folder is now gathering dust at the back of a cupboard.

'It's only a delay. I'll keep working on the SAFE program. I can't let Pete down. I can't go back now.' I tell myself over the following weeks. I'm still running group stalls to promote the charity, yet my heart isn't in it. One evening David and me are relaxing in the garden.

'I'm giving up my self-help group.'

'Why?' David asks.

'Since I started the SAFE program and stopped self-injury, it's increasingly difficult to listen to others in pain, especially involving self-injury.'

'You know I'll support you whatever you decide.' David hugs me. Together we sit watching the sun setting. I'm now redefining myself. For years I hid behind the label of self-injurer. My search for freedom and peace has taken a new lease of life. As the Summer draws to a close, for the first time in many years, I have definite aims.

'I want to be well, to get back to work. I have a new life now I'm free of self-injury,' I announce to David.

'You'd better start looking for work then. Be careful. I don't want to see you down again.'

Back at the centre, Tony too has good advice for me. 'You're making good progress Jo, but your paintings often seem dreamlike. Are you keeping a balance?'

'What do you mean?'

'It's good to have dreams. You also need to keep events in perspective. Keep both feet on the ground.

Keeping a balance

Like many self-injurers I've thought in absolute, or black and white terms. I make a mistake, I'm a failure! Every mistake or error I made I judged myself harshly for. It takes time but we can learn to start forgiving ourselves for our human mistakes. We can be kind and gentle to ourselves, as we would be to others. To have a dream to reach for is a wonderful thing, to take small steps to making that dream a reality is how miracles happen. Keeping a daily diary of small goals and achievements is helpful. It's also important to look at the whole of our life, physical, emotional, spiritual. Do you take regular exercise? Eat healthily? Take time out to relax? Time to share with others? Do you have support form a local church or find peace in nature?

After searching for work for a few weeks I decide to phone the home where I used to work.

'Good luck,' David said. 'If you do manage to get work, it'll keep you busy when I'm away.'

'It's not long now is it?' I try not to let my fear show.

'Only five weeks until my two week training course.'

The next day I phone my boss at the home. Following a meeting with her it's arranged that I will return to work for two days a week to start. The first day at work, I'm relieved to be greeted with wide smiles.

'It's great to have you back Jo.'

'We've missed you.'

'When are you coming back full time?

'I'm so excited to be back. I've missed you all too.'

'When full time Jo?'

'I don't know yet.'

I accept now it's better to make a slow, full recovery than to rush into things. Remembering Tony's advice to keep a balance, I continue attending the centre on days off. Working and the centre fills my time. I'm so busy, I've almost forgotten David's two weeks away.'

'It's next week I go away, can you get my suit dry cleaned?' David's excitement about his training course clashes with the terror I feel inside.

'I'll take your suit in tomorrow.'

'Will you be okay Jo? David picks up on my anxiety.

'I'll be fine. You're not away for long. I'll be busy cleaning and I'll phone Sadie and Angela.'

The first two days David's away I run home, eager for his phone calls.

'Everything's going well, a lot of hard work, loads of new ideas. How's things with you?'

'I'm fine, meeting Judy and Sadie after the centre tomorrow evening.'

'I miss you Jo, take care.' Phone bleeps.

First cool Autumn breeze, I shuffle through neat piles of leaves on my way to meet Angela and Sadie for coffee. Happy memories put lightness in my step. When I was young, I remember jumping into leaves Dad had carefully raked. We laughed together. Mum made us hot chocolate and home-baked biscuits. Beginning to remember happier memories is a new positive start for me.

'You're looking well Jo,' Sadie remarks to me over steaming mugs of coffee.

'You back full time yet?' Angela asks.

'No, I'm not ready yet.'

'Doesn't usually take you this long Jo, you used to be back at work the next day after one of your escapades.'

'I need a bit more time. Tell me your news.'

I don't bother to try to explain that this time it's different. No more roller-coaster ride of elation and despair. My self-injury life

94

made up of highs of secrets, deceit, the lows of broken promises, pain and rejection.

I'm throwing my coat on the chair at home as the phone rings.

'Jo... Jo, you all right?'

'Yes, I'm okay. What's wrong?' I can't understand the fear in my mother's voice.

'Jo, David phoned me. You weren't in. Then Mrs. Dee from across the way saw you heading towards the shops.'

'Mum I'm fine. I went to meet friends. David knew I'd be late tonight.' I sigh as I put the phone down.

> You don't believe me,
> I know you don't believe me, why should you?
> Years of broken promises, false hopes and dreams.
> I'm living now, I believe in me... You can too.
> I've been through the hell of despair, pain and shame.
> Years of excuses, I looked for someone to blame.
> I know you don't believe me that I've changed.
> I know I'm different. In time maybe you too will...
> Believe me?

My second week back at work, I'm asked to do an extra shift. Eager to please I agree. By Thursday, when I get to the centre I'm exhausted. Being off sick for several months, settling into a routine of work and still working on the SAFE program is taking its toll.

'Jo,' June calls me. 'You missed your aromatherapy appointment.'

'I'm sorry, I meant to phone, I forgot, I was working.'

'I thought you'd agreed only two shifts a week Jo?'

'I wanted to help.'

Exhaustion, missing David and questions are too much. I sit and cry. 'I miss David.' I tell June between breaking down in floods of tears. June is patient and stays until I'm calm.

'Jo, it's all right. It's natural to miss your husband. He's back soon isn't he?'

'Saturday.'

That evening, instead of punishing myself for feeling hurt, I find comfort in painting a welcome home card for David. Friday I spend at the centre working on a new art project. I'm still looking forward to Pete's return, even though it's been a long time with no news.

Saturday morning, I'm anxiously waiting for David's train to arrive.

'Will he still love me? Need me? Want me? Questions race in my head.

'Jo, Jo.' David runs to me arms outstretched. My heart leaps as if dancing on rainbows.

<u>Summary</u>

- The decision to love - in forgiving others and ourselves we set ourselves free to make a fresh start. Forgiveness, I've found, is a process. We may need to keep forgiving, keep making that decision to forgive in order to set ourselves free.
- Keeping a balance - to have a dream or ambition is a wonderful thing. To take small steps to making those dreams reality is how miracles happen. It's important to find time to rest, both physically and emotionally. It's easy to slip back into old habits of overwork and ignoring our inner child.
- Breaking the secrecy of self-injury - writing down what happens, events, thoughts, feelings, before, during and after an episode of self-injury helps understanding. If possible, share this, talk it through with a professional or trusted friend. This, I've found, is the most helpful yet most difficult thing to do.

Chapter Ten

Sun Drops Reflect Love in Tear Drops

Over the weekend, David basks in praise from family and friends following his two weeks training.

'It was great. I enjoyed the course.' David proudly shows his parents his certificates.

'When will you hear about your promotion?'

'Tomorrow, I'm meeting my boss at ten o'clock.'

'Well-done son, we're so proud of you.'

'We'd better get home so I can get my suit ironed.'

'You mean I'll do the ironing!' I hug David, sharing his happiness.

Monday morning, David and me are back at work. After a particularly busy shift, I hurry home and throw myself into housework. I'm singing along to the radio, preparing tea, when the back door slams.

'Hi, is that you David? Tea won't be long.'

'Don't bother. I'm not hungry.' David throws his jacket down, pours a large Vodka and coke.

'What's wrong?' I reach out to hug David and withdraw sensing his anger.

'That dumb Mike got promoted, not me.'

'Why?'

'The boss said I wasn't management material. Stupid man. What does he know anyway?'

'What about your course? Your certificates?'

'Go away. Finish burning tea.'

It's a quiet evening, silence broken only by the clatter of glasses and me scraping burnt pans in the kitchen.

Days pass, an uneasy pact of no questions leads to silence. Rejection and hurt hang heavy in the air at home. My head fills with voices screaming.

Communication

During difficult times we need to be even more open with our loved ones and partners. Often, however, we back away leaving the other person alone and frightened. If you can try to make the first move to talk. I wish I had talked more with David.

At the day centre I find solace in painting. Dark, shadowy images depict the pain and fear I feel inside. I'm facing the challenge of putting my feelings into art or writing, instead of self-injury.

'You're deep in thought Jo.' Tony startles me.

'It's been a difficult weekend.'

'Life doesn't always go to plan Jo. We're no longer expecting Pete back.'

'Not coming back. Pete's not coming back.' Words repeat in my head, the voices start again.

'Never?'

'I'm sorry Jo, I can't say anymore.'

During the following weeks, David and me continue to muddle through. We're two hurting people living separate lives. At the centre I turn to Tony for help.

'Who's going to be my key nurse?'

'I'll be your temporary key nurse Jo.'

'When can I talk to you?'

'Fifteen minutes once a week.'

'It's not enough.'

'You must be patient Jo. There are lots of other people worse off.' I keep one eye on the clock as the second hand slices through my precious time with Tony.

'Just five more minutes.'

'I have to go.'

I remember as a child, waiting for Dad to rescue me from my mother's pain and torment. I waited in vain for years. Although Dad loved me, he had his own difficulties to cope with. It's taken me years to accept my past and learn to care for myself. To acknowledge that I'm falling back into a rescue trap is a painful realisation.

My fear of abandonment starts from when I was three and a half years old. My Mum was ill and I was taken into care. We were separated for three months. Since then I've feared loss, change, abandonment.

It's as if this child is stuck inside of me, three and a half years old, lost crying for mummy. My child's pain is so deep it cannot be comforted. No amount of love or attention ever seems to be enough to stop the tears. I long to break free from this.

> When I stop and listen I hear sobs of pain.
> When I stop and watch I see tears of shame.
> When I stop and touch I touch your heart...
> Only with love can we make a fresh start.

Change is possible

For years the only way I knew how to relate to people was either to be a carer to them or to seek their help. This left no room for adult relationships based on mutual trust and understanding of each other. For example it is easier for yourself and others if you can ask for support rather than rescue or help, to ask others for advice, ideas on how some difficulty may be overcome. It is equally important to forgive ourselves for mistakes and to take responsibility for our actions.

Change is a part of life, we can either go with the flow and follow a peaceful pathway, or fight against the inevitable. Change will happen, whether we embrace it with love or run, depends on how it reacts in our lives.

Another lonely evening at home, I remember when we used to go out, laugh, joke, drink with friends. Now David sits drinking alone.

'David?'

'What?'

'David, talk to me. I love you.'

'Everything I touch goes wrong.'

'Everything?'

'Work, other stuff.'

'Tell me.' I meet David's eyes, pools of pain.

'I've been hurt, rejected before. Why should you care? David shouts.

'I do care.'

'Go away.'

'Would you come and talk with Tony at the centre? Maybe he could help?'

'Maybe,' is David's reluctant reply.

To the outside world, David and me seem like any other couple. To us it seems like we've climbed to the top of a mountain and have been stranded there. At the top of mount Eiger. We're two hurting people, clinging onto the ragged rocks. Tears form to ice, pierce frail hopes. After the treacherous scramble up the shingle, last gasps of exhaustion rack troubled minds. Love is left. Love holds these two people together. Grey mist envelopes. Voices long lost carry messages of rejection and pain.

'Kill me, save me from more hurt.'
'Save me, the other pleads.'
We're two hurting people, hanging onto strands of reality.
Life's reality hits harder than hailstones that hammer down.
After endless nights of despair, hope, trust and fight have all been destroyed.
All that remains is love.
Love bonds these two people closer than any legal or metal bondage.
Lightening splits dark sky.
'Go, leave me, save yourself, for I must die.'
'Stay a while longer,' the other pleads.
Two hurting people reaching out in desperation. Acceptance will come in time.
Dawn breaks, first rays of weak sun light up shadowed faces.
Love is all that has held these two people through the turmoil.
Only love is strong enough to see them through the dark days of despair and doubt that lie ahead.
'Hold me, I'm scared.'
Tears mingle with dewdrops.

The following week, David and me have our first meeting with Tony and June at the day centre. Slowly we are learning to support and trust each other. I've been clear of self-injury for several months, yet the physical pain hasn't eased.

'My arms drive me crazy!' I cry to David over and over.

'Maybe it's the cold weather or the extra shifts you're doing?' David hugs me 'They'll get better in time.'

'I'm going to see my doctor at the surgery' I announce to David after a night of excruciating pain.

'I'm scared I'll lose my arms they hurt so badly. What have I done?' My directness stuns my doctor. He pauses for a moment, and then examines my arms.

'Why Jo?'

'I can't explain. Tell me what's wrong.' I shake inside, as I take in the doctor's words.

'Permanent... could have lost arm... minimum of ten years to heal...'

'I'm sorry Jo.' The kindly doctor pats me on the shoulder as I leave.

'It's good to see you looking so well in yourself though.'

The changing season, from Autumn to Winter, marks a change in me. Now I'm free from self-injury I'm taking risks in positive ways. I'm choosing brighter clothes, making the most of outings with David and having physiotherapy to help my arms heal. I'm now working three shifts a week. I find inspiration from the residents' courage and sense of humour. I know that to continue working I need to take care of myself. Through June's patience and aromatherapy treatments, I'm learning to listen to my body. I'm allowing myself time to relax, to allow tears. In accepting pain and sadness, I'm also free to let in happiness, laughter and fun. David and me are continuing with our meetings at the centre, talking and building trust with each other.

Life is a miracle

Did you experience a miracle today? I did, I woke up this morning and looked out. From my window I saw a new day. Fresh rainfall left grass shining in the sun. I heard birds singing. I ran out and felt damp grass beneath my feet. I had cold coffee and burnt toast for breakfast and it tasted great! Being alive after seventeen years of surviving is exciting! From age sixteen I felt confused and hurt, I wanted to shut out the pain I felt.

'If you don't feel, you die, because it is through feeling that you find meaning and purpose. If feeling is shut down you have to create excitement and pain in order to feel alive.' Quote by Chuck Spezzano, taken from book, *'Awaken the gods.'*

I survived from one crisis to another for seventeen years. Desperate to hide from myself I tried alcohol, abused medication, took stupid risks. I paid a price. Backed up against a cold, stone wall, too scared to cry. I survived. Trapped in a self-made prison. I lived on a roller-coaster ride of excitement and pain. My roller-coaster ride became faster, more dangerous, wouldn't stop. I thought I couldn't stop.

In May of this year, my roller coaster smashed to earth. I crash landed. Dirty, crying, I was broken inside. I didn't know who I was or where I was. I was past caring if I survived or died. I spent over four weeks in hospital. Nurses cared, my family stuck by me. Kindness, acceptance and love gave me hope. I felt accepted and loved. 'God gives us life one day at a time, even then in his love he gives us a night to rest before trying again,' my Gran used to say.

David and me are shopping one Saturday in the middle of November. The first signs of Christmas are out, with Advent calendars and Christmas gifts neatly stacked in village stores.

My mood seems to have fallen with the grey weather. It seems wrong to feel hurt, sad at Christmas time. Seems like the world is out partying! I keep my thoughts of self-injury hidden.

I'm still working on the SAFE program, this is helping me identify patterns and cycles to my self-injury behaviours.

Example of my cycle of self-injury behaviour

(Although the triggers are my own experience, many people may identify or recognise similar patterns.)

1. Feeling hurt or insecure.
   Example: Pete leaving, changes at work or family illness.
2. Rescue trap.
   Example: seeking to rescue my friend who is still cutting and then blaming myself for not being successful
3. Confusion, increasing emotional pain inside.
   At this point I often seek rescue for myself. With my meetings with Tony, I'm improving at being direct, but still find leaving hard and tend to cling.

4. Questions.
   Am I okay? Guilty? Bad? Can I cope on my own? I have a mixture of increasing insecurity and confusion.
5. Crisis point.
   The urge to self-injure is strong. I'm desperate to find peace and space from the screaming in my head, to stop time and pain. If I give in and self-injure I make more chaos, change, increasing rejection and guilt.

Monday morning, I've reached crisis point. I know I need to break my cycle of self-injury by caring for myself and using the SAFE program. In the afternoon I see my doctor.
   'I'm struggling, it's hard. I keep thinking about cutting.'
   'You must have reasons. Tell me what's changed.'
   'It's just memories. I hurt inside.'
   'It's normal to feel Jo.'
   'I'm still doing art, writing. I've even started writing a pantomime.' I sigh. 'It takes so long the hurt is so deep.'
   'Would you come back to the evening group Jo? I think you need support at the moment.'
   The following week I return to the evening group. I feel such relief to be accepted back amongst old friends.
   'You can choose to make today a good day. Do things you enjoy. By tomorrow you will have built happy memories.' I think on this advice for some time.
   During the following weeks when I feel stressed, exhausted from work, I'm planning the pantomime. Making props, designing scenery. Carefree moments covered in glue, paint and glitter.
   One evening David is unusually quiet, after two or three drinks he announces.
   'I've been put on a three day week for the Winter. Not enough work.'
   'You could help with the pantomime.' As soon as I've spoken, I regret my offer. Having been used to keeping a large part of my life secret due to self-injury, I find it difficult to share projects.
   The first of December, residents at the home are busy making plans for Christmas.
   'Can you do a poster for our carol singing? We need singers too, will you join us?'

'I'll do a poster. I'd better not sing. Folk pay me to move on!' We laugh together at this novel idea for fundraising.

Later that day, I'm buried under piles of pantomime props when David shouts, 'phone for you Jo.'

'This is Mr Giles, head of the health promotion unit. I'm planning a two-day promotional event for local charities early next year. Would you be interested?' I stare at the phone, willing it to disappear.

'I'm not doing much with the group now.'

'It's an ideal opportunity then. I'll put your group in.'

'I'm...'

'Good. That's settled then. Speak to you nearer the time.'

'Why didn't you just say no?' David asks.

'I tried to explain I wasn't involved with the group so much. I find it hard to say no. There's so many people in need.'

Tension builds inside me the next few weeks as I support David, work extra shifts to cover staff sickness and battle with half-finished pantomime props. Many of the residents have coughs, colds and flu and due to their disabilities these routine illnesses hit them harder than most. Caring for others in distress is triggering painful memories too. Memories of caring for my mother. Running home from school, first check if Gran is safe and well then home to mum.

Although the centre and evening group are my main support through this, I still miss Pete. One evening I write a list of all the positive things I learned from working with Pete. This is something you could do if a member of staff you trusted leaves or if you suffer bereavement. To choose to remember positive things.

My list of positive things I learned from working with Pete

1. Unconditional love heals
2. Respect for both myself and others
3. To see humour, even through difficult or painful times
4. To know that I can be a friend to myself
5. Acceptance and love heals
6. To challenge my thoughts
7. I have choice, control in my life

8.   I can face my feelings of insecurity without self-injury
9.   Believe in myself, abilities, inner strength
10.   To dream good dreams think of flying
11.   To accept and forgive myself
12.   I have a future
13.   Accept my past, including mistakes as a learning experience
14.   To celebrate good memories
15.   I have responsibility to communicate directly, honestly to people. Without resorting to self-injury.

The following week, I have a review with my doctor.

'I want to get back to full time work.' I said

'No, not yet,' my doctor firmly replies, 'I'll review work again in the new year.'

Although I'm disappointed, I understand I need to resist the temptation to set unachievable goals. The risk of returning to my life as a self-injurer is still there.

'I'm fed up!' I tell June later that week at my aromatherapy session. ' I keep fighting. It's like I'm running through quicksand.'

'It's all right Jo. You're doing well. It's okay to be tired.' In her kind patient way, June continues to build trust with me.

One week to Christmas, David and me are boxing up the last of the props for the pantomime, to be held at the centre the following day.

'Do you think it will be all right?'

'For the sixtieth time yes!' David hugs me. 'What's the worst thing that can happen?'

'I might forget something.'

'You've got two of everything!'

'Better to reject myself first.' The old voices taunt me, as I toss and turn, unable to sleep.

'Mother Goose ate the golden egg!' packs the community room with laughter, fun and music.

Mistakes such as me playing the backing music to 'The twelve days of Christmas', while the cast sing 'Rudolph the red noised reindeer' only add to the fun. I'm delighted to have found a creative outlet for my energy.

The next few days pass in a whirl of work and Christmas shopping for David and me. We invite friends and family to join us for Christmas day. The holidays are a happy time for David and me. New year's eve I snuggle up to David, watching pictures flicker in the roaring log fire.

'It's nearly midnight. Any New Year resolutions Jo?'

'To be with you forever.'

New year's day, I'm up at daybreak. I walk barefoot across our frosted lawn. A beautiful day, a fresh start. In the distance, doors crash as the last partygoers arrive home. In the corner of the garden a splash of red catches my eye.

'Poor little robin.' I scoop the tiny bird in my hands carry him indoors. The sun is breaking through as I hold the still, cold robin up to the window.

'Gran will love you,' I whisper. 'I'm sorry.'

A single silent tear drops to the floor, as sun drops of painful memories reflect in teardrops.

Summary

- Change is possible - both to change from a life of survival of self-injury and how we relate to other people. This takes time, please be patient, and praise every effort you make.
- Life is a miracle - just by being alive you are a miracle, unique, special. You are a wonderful person just as you are. Even if you don't feel like it!
- Understanding of our patterns of self-injury helps in breaking the cycle. Once you are aware of triggers it is possible to intervene and stop from self-injury.
- Unconditional love and acceptance heals. Once we can truly accept ourselves as we are, then we are halfway to improving our situation.
- Recovery from relapse takes time. Try to focus on positive things, find one positive thought, one positive action, one positive feeling. Make a list of happy memories.
- Learning to love and accept our inner child - our inner child is always there, sometimes happy, sometimes sad. Learn to give our child a hug e.g. hug arms around yourself, watch a

comedy video, have a bubble bath, play with animals, pray, sing, play music, relaxation, aromatherapy.

Chapter Eleven

Dancing in Sun Drops

A new year, a fresh start. With David still working part-time hours, I'm determined to increase my hours at work. I need to do this both for financial security and to increase my self-esteem. It's a few weeks into the New Year before I find time to see Tony at the centre.

'New year Jo, what are your plans?'

'To get back to work full time.'

'Have you thought about leaving the centre?' It's a few moments before I can find words. Cold fear drips, my hands are suddenly clammy.

'Maybe I could leave in June. I'll have been clear of self-injury for a year then.' Although a program of time and dependency reduction at the centre is agreed with me, terror grips me inside. Changes threaten my security.

'You okay with these arrangements then Jo?' Tony's voice breaks my thoughts.

'I'm scared of leaving. I'll miss you.'

'Jo, we're setting you free, not rejecting you. For everyone there's a time to move on.'

During the next week, I arrange to work full-time for six weeks as a trial basis to return to full time contract hours at the home.

One evening I'm relaxing with David when the phone rings. 'Hello this is Mr. Giles, remember the health promotion event?'

'Mmm yes.' As the phone crackles I rack my mind to remember... the group charity promotion... two-day event... new year...

'It's all booked. I'm sure you have all your group information ready to do displays.'

'I'll be ready.' I promise.

'I'll phone the evening before to confirm start times.' I sink back onto the sofa, cuddle up to David.

'That was about the charity promotion. I'll sort it out later.'

'Don't forget Jo.'

The next weeks fly past, I'm busy working, visiting my parents, trying to support David who has yet another job refusal. My shifts at work are increasingly busy. Often the first time I stop to have a break is at handover time for the next shift.

'It's the end of my six weeks trial next week.' I remind my supervisor at work.

'You've done well Jo. If you're finding things too much tell someone though.'

'I'm fine.' I insist. Inside I'm crying.

At the art therapy group, my tears mingle with splashes of blue and black paint.

'You having a hard time Jo?' Tony asks.

'I don't want to leave the centre. I feel rejected, pushed out into the cold.'

'Jo, you're not being pushed out, but set free. Look at your long-term goals. See this as a beginning.'

Planning for a future

Having achieved some time free from self-injury, the time has come to look forward. The future can seem frightening if we look too far ahead. It is helpful to plan small achievable goals. Plan one goal for each month for the next six months. This could be something physical like joining a gym, or something practical like seeking financial advice. It's not the effort of starting a new project that I find hard, it's keeping level. After years of success then crash, failure of self-injury, it's difficult to learn a new way of living.

Later that evening David and me are walking by the sea front.

'Come on Jo, what's bothering you?'

'Mary my favourite resident at work is really ill. She's such a brave and beautiful lady. It breaks my heart to see her in pain. I have to leave the day centre. I haven't been able to see my boss yet to know if I've passed my six weeks trial.'

'Slow down Jo, there's no need to get so worked up.'

'You don't understand!' I snap, turn away to hide my tears of rage and hurt.

'Be good, don't cry.' Voices echo in my head.

'Let's go home, I'll make coffee.' David hugs me.

The following day David is waiting for me when I return home from work.

'I've got a surprise for you Jo. We're off to St. Malo at the weekend.'

'David, that's wonderful.' The rest of the evening passes in happy hunting for passports and maps. As David packs our cases on Friday evening I sit alone in the kitchen.

'What's wrong Jo? I thought you'd be packed before me.'

'I'm tired.' I said. Inside my head voices scream, 'CUT! RUN! You're bad, you're useless. You don't deserve nice things.'

Thankfully by the time we arrive in St. Malo the voices have ceased. The weekend passes quickly in a rush of blustery sea walks, hot crunchy baguettes and cool wine.

Tuesday morning we're both back at work. It's another difficult shift for me, with six of the ten residents in bed with colds and flu. Mary, my favourite resident has complications. The doctor is called. At handover at the end of the shift we are informed that Mary has died peacefully. I run home and cry. I cry until I have no tears left.

On my next day off I attend the day centre. I'm sitting having coffee when I glance towards the office, Pete is in the office. Pete, my former key nurse is back. A whirl of emotions floods over me.

'How can he just turn up like that? Why did he leave me before?'

'Hello Pete.'

'You're looking well Jo,' the phone ringing interrupts further conversation.

'See you later.' I leave, grateful to escape.

As I wander home, I remember my mother leaving suddenly then returning months later. As I was only four years old I didn't understand that mummy was ill.

The inner child

We all have an inner sense of fun, our sense of childhood that never dies. Also within us, because of past hurts, our inner child may cry out in pain at times. It is important to try to listen to these cries, to accept them as our needs. At times we need to stop and give ourselves space and permission to cry, to play music, to go with our feelings. Accepting our feelings breaks their intensity. Instead of adding guilt to our original feeling e.g. I feel angry, I'm a bad person for feeling angry. Accepting our feelings is a more peaceful way to live. Relaxation, deep breathing is also helpful if you have intense feelings or anxiety.

As an adult, I now understand that my mother suffered too as a result of our separation. She too watched for hours out of dull windows at a grey sky, wondering if I was happy or sad.

I regret not welcoming Pete back, through a mist of tears late evening I write this poem...

To dream good dreams

To dream good dreams, think of flying, you said the day you left.
I tried, even flew Concorde! I did my best.
My planes all crashed, shards of pain. I had no rest.
Some advice! I thought, yet I cried when you left.
Dream good dreams, think of flying, I want to be free.
I searched, begged for rescue, but only I had the key.
Through pain, torment, I remembered your words.
Acceptance, love helped set me free.
My best dream came true; you're back once more.
I wanted to hug you when you walked through the door,
My plans all went wrong, and now I just long...
To thank you, for I'm finding where I belong...
Is not in the pits of shame and despair...
But up where rainbows fill the air.

Desperate to stay positive, I throw myself into work, writing and art. I also spring clean the house.

'You okay Jo?' David leaps out of the way of the hoover.

'I'm fine. Just the attic to clean now.'

'Jo, slow down it's your weekend off.'

Finally the hoover whines to a stop. I lean against the kitchen door.

'You don't understand! I've got extra shifts at work next week. There's Mum and Dad to take shopping and your parents to visit.

The following week is as I predicted, busy. Doctors and ambulances call regularly at the home, filling the air with fear and tension.

'Can you stay another hour Jo?'

'Can you change your day off?' I sigh, down another cold coffee.

'I must be good, quiet. You're guilty, bad.' Voices start again in my head.

Friday morning it's unusually quiet at work. For me there's no peace. Inside my head is filled with voices screaming.

'What's up Jo? You're quiet today.'

'Careful Jo, I thought you'd fall then.'

'That was a straight transfer. What's up?' Questions I feel unable to answer.

'I need to go.' My whole body shakes as I talk to my supervisor.

'Take care Jo. Go and see your doctor.'

Through a blur of tears and fear, staff at the centre, then the duty doctor talk gently to me.

'We're admitting you to the ward Jo.'

For three or four hours I cling to the same chair in the smoking lounge. I rock. I cry. I'm too scared to move. People come and go, I sit, gripped by fear. Screaming fills me inside.

'You feeling any better Jo?' A nurse sits, holds my hand. 'It's okay, you're safe here. Talk to us when you're ready.'

Sunday morning I find a member of staff to talk to.

'Do you want to tell me what's happened to make you feel so bad?'

'I've been scared of losing people... alot of illness at work.' The nurse waits patiently as I cry. 'It's not just that, I've been taking myself to breaking point over the last six weeks. This time I haven't been able to get back on my feet.'

'You haven't cut Jo, that's real progress.'

'How I felt Friday, scared, desperate, that's how I used to feel before I cut.'

'Is there anything else worrying you?'

'I hurt someone...' I look away. 'I'd better go.' My thoughts race as I walk away. I hurt Pete. I'm letting David down by being here.

Monday morning I ask to see the doctor.

'I want to be discharged.'

'You sure you're okay Jo?'

'I'll be fine.' I said. I need to be... David needs me.

The next day I phone my boss at work and apologise for leaving on Friday.

'We need to talk to you Jo.' My boss said.

'Can it keep until Monday? I've got the charity promotion on this week.'

'Nine o'clock Monday then.'

Sitting in the village hall, listening to speakers on self-injury, my gaze wanders. A teenage girl sits, picking bandaged arms. My instinct is to run over, to hug her, to tell her it does get easier.

During the coffee break, I'm handing out leaflets, I see the girl standing to one side.

'Can I help?'

'I doubt it. No-one can help.'

'I felt like that once too. You're not alone, here's the group phone number. I haven't got a magic answer, but if you'd like to talk I'll listen.'

'Sometimes I hurt so much I can't put it into words.'

'Sometimes it seems easier to self-harm than to find words.' I reply.

'You understand then?'

'I'm here to listen. Here's a list of crisis phone numbers too.' I hand the girl leaflets as the next speaker walks to the stage.

You are not alone

Self-injury is a lonely way to live. There are crisis phone lines, self-help groups and information available via the Internet. You may feel alone, like you are the only one in the world who self-injures. There are a lot of us! We get scared too, but you can still find help and support.

By the end of the two-day event I feel exhausted. In the evening I fall onto the settee next to David.

'I've got full time hours, starting Monday.' David said.

'That's great. We'll be able to save and have a holiday.'

'I'm not sure if I want to do full time, my parents need extra help now, especially after Dad's recent fall.

'Everything will be okay. We're together, that's all that matters.' I hug David close.

The phone shrills into the quietness. 'Jo, it's Mum. Aunt Amy has been taken ill. She's in hospital. Can you run me and Dad up to visit in the morning?'

The weekend passes in a blur of shopping and driving our parents round to various appointments. Sunday evening I curl up to David, comforted by his warmth.

'Its tomorrow you see your boss isn't it?'

I have a difficult decision to make. Should I go on pushing myself to the limit, to care for my family and caring at work? Or give up the job I love? It's a question that leaves me tossing and turning long after David is snoring.

In my efforts to be free, to dance in sun drops, I'm taking myself to breaking point. Is this a final scream of pain as I spiral back to a life of self-injury?

Summary

- We need to accept and cherish our inner child. Also to accept that at times memories may be upsetting and we need to go with our feelings and be kind to ourselves.
- Hold onto our dreams, however impossible they may seem. To have a dream, to make even tiny steps to making that dream a reality is giving our lives hope and meaning.
- Keep on a level, try to maintain a balance of work and play. To make time to relax and enjoy life.

Chapter Twelve

Without night sky there are no stars,
Without feeling… no life

Monday morning, bleary eyed I slam my hand out.
'Stupid alarm…stop!'
'It's the phone.'
'Hello… oh Mum. I'm sorry. I'm wide-awake now. Blissful escape of sleep lost.
'Aunt Amy died last night.' Finding little consolation in burnt toast and cold coffee, I hurry to meet my boss.
'Sorry I'm late Jo. You know what Monday mornings are like.' I shuffle awkwardly into the office.
'I can't work here anymore. I'm sorry.' I said.
'Why? You're a good worker Jo. I thought you were over your difficulties.'
'I'm sorry, I need a break, a different job.' I choke back tears as I run home. Once home I scan the local paper. No time to cry for Aunt Amy or the job I loved so much. Over the next week I phone every situation vacant advert.
'Sorry, already taken.'
'No experience.'
'Why did you leave your last job?' So many ways to say NO! Evenings, David and me hold each other tight. We're two hurting people, clinging together through stormy nights and troubled times.
'I'm scared, my dad isn't well.' I said.
'My mum's going into hospital tomorrow for tests,' David replies.
'I'm sorry. I'm not even earning any money. I'm useless!'
'Come on Jo. You can't give in, why don't you visit the centre?'
'I'm sorry. I love you David.'
I shuffle, rub my scars, look anxiously at my doctor, then Tony.
'Please…can I stay on at the centre? I'll get part-time work.'
'You can do full time now Jo. Come to the evening group.'
'I'm scared… to be alone… to fall.'
'It's time to move on Jo.' My doctor stands as he speaks.
'Pete? Is he coming back?'

'No, at least not in the foreseeable future. It's time to make a fresh start.' Tony stands to see me out.

'See you at the evening group,' my doctor shouts as I slam the office door.

That evening I shut out most of the group discussion, staring out of the window preferable to owning my feelings of anger and pain. One bit of advice penetrates my defences. 'The best way to honour the dead is to keep working.' Aunt Amy was a fighter. The last thought I have as I fall asleep is to keep fighting.

Remembering loved ones

We are all certain to experience loss of loved ones during our lives and it is natural and appropriate to grieve their loss. At some point it may be helpful to think of the loved one and ask what they would like us to do. For myself, I've always been sure that Gran would like me to do my best at work and to care for my family. By continuing to live, we are celebrating their memories rather than being drowned in a sea of sorrow and loss.

The following morning after David has left for work, I clean the house, weed the garden and bake cakes for David. Glass sparkles, wood gleams, I've even scrubbed the front doorstep. Six o'clock, I arrange flowers and set the tea ready.

'Wow, cherry cake.' David mumbles through chunks of cake. 'Any luck in getting work?'

'Not yet, I've phoned three more. The grocery store is supposed to phone back. I don't suppose they'll bother.'

In the early hours of the morning I listen to David snoring, my mind racing, my body screaming for sleep. I wanted so much to keep my job at the home, to help others in need... I feel I've let the residents down by leaving. Yet my parents and David's needs must surely come first? I pace the silent house, walk out into cold night air. I stare up at the stars searching for inspiration. Finding nothing I return to bed.

The next morning my head is filled with voices screaming for attention, I abandon my search for work for the day and head for the day centre.

'I need to talk to Tony.'

'Tony's not in today, do you want to talk to me?' I stare up into deep blue eyes. 'I'm Matthew, I'm here for a few weeks to cover staff holidays.'

'Okay.' We sit in the quiet room. I wipe my hands on my jeans, sweat drips.

'What's bothering you Jo?' Matthew leans forward.

'I want to self-harm.'

'What are your feelings Jo?'

'I really want to self-harm. I don't know why I'm bothering talking to you.'

'Jo, there's a difference between your urge to self-harm and your feelings. Tell me what's happening to upset you.'

'I've left my job. It mattered a lot to me. I really cared about the folks I was nursing.'

'Why did you leave Jo?'

'I had to, I was feeling burnt out. I'm trying to support David, my husband. He gets depressed too you see. Then my parents need more care now they're older.'

'You'll soon find another job.'

'The folks were my family. I needed them.'

'So change is difficult for you?'

'I need people to stay the same, not to leave. When people leave, or die, or when I leave I feel abandoned.'

'Abandoned?'

'It's like I'm a child again. I'm trapped all over again. It's stupid…'

'Take your time Jo, it's okay.'

I was only three. I tried to be brave. I tried not to cry, but I was scared. I was looking for mummy but I couldn't find her.'

'What happened to your mum?'

'She was very ill, someone took her to hospital. I know now she went to a psychiatric hospital for treatment for severe depression. I was only little. The people at the home I was taken to said not to cry. I learned from then to keep my feelings inside.' I'm rocking in my chair now, biting my hand. I can't cry.

'Thank you for trusting me.' Matthew said softly. 'Can you trust me enough to share your pain with me?'

'I was only three. I had a pink rabbit with me, but I missed my Mum…' tears splash over me now, my body shakes with pain. I cry for my inner child who was lost. I cry for my mother. I cry for myself. Matthew stays, his gentle voice soothing.

Healing the inner child

Matthew's support in listening and accepting me helped me to see myself as a whole person. I understand now that my self-injury has been about separating parts of myself e.g. child, judge, weak adult, dreamer. When I self-injure the judge punishes the child. By accepting my child I become whole, so there is less need to self-injure.

Once we begin the journey of healing we take control of our lives, by making decisions. Decisions to let memories rest in the past and focus on the present moment. We decide to care for ourselves and raise our self-esteem, to accept and nurture our inner child.

Late Friday afternoon, David calls me to the phone.
'Yes okay… I'll see you Monday morning then.'
'I've got a job.' I whirl round the kitchen with David.
'Where? When do you start?'
'The grocery store, Monday morning.'
I throw myself into my new work, eagerly stacking shelves with Easter eggs and novelties.
'You're doing okay' the boss said, 'We're closed over Easter, so see you Tuesday.'
Good Friday morning, David and me are baking cakes and hot cross buns for family and friends.
'Mum always bakes extra for friends…' I smile 'I used to bash the Christmas puddings with a wooden spoon.'
'Bet that helped a lot!' David laughs with me. The Easter holidays pass happily for us. On my last day at the centre, Tony gives me one last piece of advice.
'Remember life is never perfect. It's a journey. Live in the moment. Make one change at a time.'
At the evening group, I'm eager to share my news.

'I've started a new job, and left the centre. Things are on the up.'

'It's good to see you so happy Jo.'

<u>Celebrating the inner child</u>

A lot of my fight has been to block out my child inside. By blocking pain, anger, hurt, all feelings are blocked. By allowing tears and sad memories, I'm also remembering happy times. Birthday parties, Mum baking bread, Dad teaching me how to draw and paint. To feel whole, we need to integrate our inner child. This can be done slowly, imagine holding your child's hand while out walking. Do something that is fun… read a children's book, eat ice-cream and visit the park or beach. Spend time with young children or animals.

During the weeks that follow, I'm busy trying out new projects, challenging my insecurity surrounding change in fun ways. Evenings find me buried under library books, boxes of art materials and papers. Weekends I help David in the garden. On my day off I search the shops for something to buy for his birthday on Sunday. I struggle home with a large model aircraft kit. As David is called into work, I spend Sunday morning decorating our lounge. Balloons, streamers, posters, ribbons adorn every wall. I bake a huge cake decorated with model aircraft. I remember my childhood birthdays. Mum always baked a cake, even when she wasn't feeling well.

After tea, Mum and me leave David chatting with the other guests to make coffee.

'Remember Sunday teas at Gran's?'

'How could we ever forget?' Mum smiles. 'Especially Gran's ninetieth birthday party. You bought a huge pink cake decorated with pink roses. Gran was so happy and proud to be with all of her family.'

Slowly I'm healing, remembering happy times and seeing my life in perspective. I accept my parents loved and cared for me. I remember Mum teaching me to read, the precious gift of learning and escape into books.

Almost a year has passed now since I said goodbye to my life of self-injury. So much has changed. Last night my father's sister died, awakening painful feelings for me. Loss sparks fears of abandonment. It's always my fear that if one family member dies others will follow.

Choosing to live

There will always be difficult days, challenges to face in our lives. People will move on, perhaps leaving us behind. There will always be other people to love, new friends to make. We will find fresh ideas, new experiences. Try to remember those who have been kind to you, the nurse who cared enough to listen, the friend who stayed, the doctor who asked why? If there is only one person who cared for you, that is reason enough to live. If you can think of one person you can help that too is a good reason to live.

I know I must keep going, keep pushing through my insecurity. At my next meeting with my doctor I discuss my plans to move on. Through talking with my doctor, these are the things I now understand about my difficulties with leaving. I feel the need to initiate leaving anywhere so I don't feel abandoned when other people leave. It's also about feeling in control and having a choice.

1. The pattern I used to follow was feeling threatened by changes or leaving. My intense fear and insecurity led me to cling to others. I would then blame myself and add guilt and anger to my feelings of fear. I'd often try to spark anger in others, then I could justify my own anger and leave fuelled by anger. I also used anger as a way of masking hurt.
2. I cling to find love and comfort. I'm scared I could drown in my own sadness. If I expressed my anger it may destroy others. I'm learning to sit with my feelings. To know I can live and feel safely.
3. I'm ashamed at my desire to cling. Deeply ashamed and guilty at even admitting my cravings to be loved and held.

Later that day I attend the evening group. 'Is it okay to talk about leaving without giving a definite date?'

'Of course it's okay Jo.'

'Whenever I talk about leaving it's scary, painful. I think about self-injury to stop my feelings. It's a constant battle raging inside. I want to be free, but I'm still scared to let my feelings out.'

Midnight, I sit on the garden wall, alone. I'm exhausted, past even finding solace in the beautiful night sky. For over an hour at the group I talked and then cried as if my heart would break.

I finally have some understanding of how my mother became ill and how much she loved me. The way I understand it now is, that my mother had eight years of heaven, being loved by her Mum, my Gran. Then five years of hell being separated during the war years. When my mother became ill, she tried to protect me. Events beyond her control meant that we were separated for a time. Mother never stopped loving me. Another painful yet healing thought is that my mother tried to hold me close, to protect me from the terror she experienced as a child. In order to save me from ever being taken away again we had an unusually close relationship. This tight bond, however, made it difficult for me to separate my feelings from my mothers.

A lot of my fight for freedom has involved me lashing out in anger, often inappropriately, frequently at myself. At last, after years of searching I'm finding peace and forgiveness. The last thought I hold as I drift to sleep is that love heals.

Love is...

Love is compassionate, gentle in touch. Love is staying even when you don't understand the situation. Love is asking why and listening to the answer. Love is touching another's scars. Love is acceptance.

Loving yourself is about accepting all of yourself. Celebrating your uniqueness. Love is giving yourself rewards and treats.

Love is a great big hug.

The next day at work, although exhausted from little sleep, I feel calm. Following a hot, busy afternoon I'm grateful for a light breeze on the way home. Shutting out the roar of traffic, I'm lost in my own thoughts. Almost full circle now, I'm breaking free. One-year self-injury free. At the start of my journey I blamed others. I pause, look up at the huge oak tree whose branches seem to be sweeping heaven's door. I hated this world for not making my dreams come true. Now I'm taking responsibility for making my own dreams happen. Almost home, I can smell a barbeque cooking.

'Happy birthday Jo.' David runs out, hugs me covering me with smuts of smoke. 'Thought I'd surprise you.'

'It's a wonderful surprise.' I whirl David round, laughing until dizzy, we fall onto damp grass. During the evening we chatter with our parents over burnt sausages and iced drinks. Late evening I wander off for a moment to watch the sun setting. I know I'm far from perfect. I Accept that I still have painful memories, that loss, change are still difficult issues.

Midnight passes, David and me stand outside, holding each other. Pure white moon, dark silk skies, stars flicker.

'So many changes over the last year.'

'We're still together, holding on in love.'

Summary

- We need to try to honour the memory of those we have lost, to carry on working. To carry on with the small acts of kindness that remind us of their lives. Baking for ourselves or others, feeding the birds, giving someone a smile. In this way we keep their memory alive.
- Healing the inner child, by taking time to enjoy life. To walk to the park or beach, to rent a comedy video, to eat ice-cream. To let ourselves have and experience feelings.
- Relapse - if you have self-injured after a period of time free from self-injury it's easy to feel a failure. We need to remember that life is a journey, a learning curve. Mistakes are opportunities to learn. If you have self-harmed, remember you are still a special, unique person. You are still valuable, loveable. Your self-injury may feel painful and upsetting, it does not make you bad. Please be kind to yourself, you have hurt yourself enough, it is time to begin

again. If you are admitted to hospital the following may be helpful,

- Try to be honest with staff, to build trust.
- Take small steps, negotiate time out from the ward slowly
- Praise every effort, even if you don't reach your goal, you tried.
- Choosing to live, every day to make the choice to feel and to make the best of the day. We can choose to see events as challenges or adventures rather than as disasters. Change is inevitable it's how we see and react to change that is important. Keep building your self-esteem, remind yourself of all the times you have coped. If you do have a set back that is all it is… a learning experience.

Because I could never thank you enough
I choose each day to live, to love.
Because you helped me see I have a choice,
To live or survive,
Today I choose to live, to love.
Thank you.
Love sets me free to love.

Appendix I

Art Therapy

Art therapy is sometimes referred to as a 'triangular relationship' because it adds to the relationship between a client and a therapist a third element: the art images produced by the client. These images, produced within a safe containment of a therapeutic alliance are empowered and meaningful. They are often also beautiful, but their beauty is not to be judged by conventional standards: they may be lyrical, wistful, raw, stark, painful, angry, joyous, emancipatory. They embody the feelings and experiences of the client, often in ways which cannot be expressed in words. In this, they form a bridge upon which the client and therapist may meet in order to construct the therapeutic encounter from which healing arises.

When art therapy is conducted in a group setting, this triangular relationship is expanded into multiple dimensions. The group becomes a crystal in whose facets the multiple images are reflected, and reflected again. It becomes an intimate community whose members generate therapeutic meanings with and for each other (Waller, 1993). The art therapy group which I am privileged to facilitate – and of which Jo, the author of this book, is a member – seeks to to uphold such a culture. The group members explore, affirm, enquire interpret and sometimes challenge. The art images, held at the heart of the group's working, radiate their light and their darkness. Sometimes, through discussion, they yield meanings unconsciously embodied (Schaverien, 1992). Sometimes they are accepted in silence, their colours and forms allowed to speak for themselves. Always, the group is a space of respect and mutual support – a place where creativity and humanity of persons who may have suffered negation and rejection might find acceptance, affirmation and healing.

Gary A. Ayres
February 2003

References

Schaverien, J (1992) *The revealing image: analytical art psychotherapy in theory and practice.* London: Routledge

Waller, D (1993) *Group interactive art therapy: its use in training and treatment.* London: Routledge

Appendix II

Group Therapy for Self-Harm

A useful way to look at those who harm themselves is to regard the people as having a conflict within their selves. We can conceive of our inner selves as possessing multiple potential roles that can act as if autonomously and sometimes antagonistically against one another, often apparently independent from our conscious observing and executive self (or "I"). This is most evident when the sub-selves (the "me") are activated by anxieties, triggered from outside ourselves, and thrown into disequilibrium. The struggling inner system then requires control and balance. We can refer to this multifaceted self as our inner family, made up of what can be termed roles, parts, or sub-systems.

The "I" f each of us can be regarded as our personal and individual therapist, with the task of helping the inner parts to understand their roles in relationship to each other and to the "I". With this comprehension comes a reconciliation and a working together to maintain the integrity of the parts of the self as a whole, in harmony and under the operation of the "I". This is the private, inner group.

There are three other groups to which this internal family system relates. The original group is the family-of-origin of the individual subject: the parents, siblings and, to varying degrees, members of the extended family. The pattern of interactions during childhood plays a large part in shaping the internal family system of later life, and their influence upon the subject remains, whether or not the real family members are alive and in direct contact with the subject.

The second family system comprises the significant people currently in the life of the self-harming person. They may still comprise some of the original family members, but included any "new" family, such as spouse, partner, friends, work colleagues and important social figures.

Finally, in a therapy group, there is the third family or system to which the subject relates outwardly. As the group develops, relationships between the members are affected by the interactions of the internal family systems of each individual. Some of these interactions are themselves influenced by the historical and developmental influences upon the sub-selves. Others are influenced by people and events in the current life of the members outside the group.

The task of the group is to enable the relationship between the members to develop. When this process becomes obstructed, it is function of the group to examine the sources of the difficulties. They become manifest in the types of interaction within the therapy group, and these in turn can be understood by examining the internal system or sub-group of each member, assisted by an ongoing examination of the influences of the original family, and of current, real life, family and social groups.

The method by which a therapy group performs its task is to experience itself as like a family system and (what natural and internal family systems are unable to do) reflect upon this experience from the viewpoint of the group itself, and of each of its members.

The function of the therapist is primarily to help the group keep to its task. Like the "I" of an individual person, the therapist has an observing and executive role. The therapist, also being a part of the system, must reflect upon the roles taken by each member, by the group as a whole, and the part played by the therapist. In maintaining both an observing and an enabling stance – involved, yet at the same time retaining some detachment – the therapist encourages the group to keep its task without the therapist getting "lost" in the interlocking system. The therapist must think while feeling, separating one function from the other, and use this process to assist the group members also to differentiate their own thoughts from their feelings.

The primary method of achieving this task is to attend to the boundaries of the group, such as the time frame, continuity, issues of commitment to membership and to the process of putting feelings into thoughts.

This group process that applies to those who self-harm is the same as for those who attend for many other emotional and interpersonal problems. However, it will be helpful to illustrate how group therapy might operate with the person whose major problem is self-harm.

One of the inner parts of the "me", of which the conscious subject is usually only partially aware, maybe the perpetrator of self-harm, e.g., self-injury, such as cutting. From what other inner part comes the motivation to cut? One that desires to punish, to seek to control, or to anaesthetise – as by distraction – another part? What of the part that is the target of the cutting? A victim, to allow the rage of the self-harmer to be released? A child part, to be harshly trained not to have unacceptable wishes or impulses (the harming part being a stern parent or conscience)? Is the recipient part of the self-injury one that tries to avoid emotional pain, such as a sense of rejection, by becoming distant and cut off from the "I"? Is the cutting part a disguised "rescuer", bringing the "I" back into contact with reality by the physical pain of the cutting?

Why cannot the "I" see the "us", the inner parts that make up the "me", and check the inner self-sabotage? The parts have become split off from the "I" to protect it from what they believe to be intolerable feelings, such as helplessness: they do not think that the "I" can effectively manage their disharmony. The task of the therapy group is to help the "I" get back on track.

Consider how the corresponding roles might manifest themselves in the group. One member may present the role of group saboteur – not, obviously, by cutting someone, but by "cutting off" from the group. This may be by way of avoiding provocative or challenging encounters with other members, or by flouting group norms or rules, as by "acting-out" instead of permitting the self to feel and expressing feelings in words. "Acting-out" could be arriving late, missing sessions, or even walking out.

Another group member may present their "victim" part, and draw to itself the group's attention: such a role might be to protect one of the other group members from the perceived anger of other members, for an infringement of the group rules, such as having been verbally abusive. From a group perspective, the "victim" deflects the fire on to their self, e.g., by accepting blame too readily for some misfortune or malfunctioning of the group. Such a "victim" part may itself "act-out", e.g., walk out, change the subject, interrupt, charm, or ingratiate itself, if it senses that someone in the group is at risk or attack or of rejection. If the rest of the group colludes in this victimisation, the "victim" becomes a "scapegoat".

The task the group members then would be to restore the boundary, contain the anxiety, "see" what is covertly taking place within the group (its members and, if possible, their inner parts), and share their understanding with the rest of the group. It might then become clear that the self-harmer is operating in the group therapy context something equivalent, though disguised, to what is happening between the sub-selves of the subject. The problem may have been that, for historical reasons, the subject (the self-harmer) may have thought that blame or rejection is unbearable and therefore, by seeking to avoid it, fail to realise that it is tolerable after all – to their own self and to the other group members.

The self-directed "rage" of the self-harmer may be misconstrued; it may be a mistaken attempt to protect, much as a parent might smack a child in the belief that this is the best training to avoid danger (like crossing a busy road on its own). Alternatively, the parent's anger might be an inappropriate way of dealing with their own fear, or guilt, over not foreseeing an earlier risk of an accident to the infant. The cut off (emotionally detached) "victim" part of the self-harmer may have switched the conversation to a more comfortable subject by getting an "avoider" back on track.

However, the group process, if operating effectively, should in time reveal that the avoided topic or emotion is not unbearable, to the self-harmer, nor to the other group members, as was feared. Moreover, addressing the need to adhere to the group norms would have made the infliction of physical harm unnecessary.

The process of the group therapy in this way allows the internal parts of each member to interact with the internal parts of the other group members. The observing and executive "I" of each member participates with the "I" of each of the other group members in the context of containing boundary maintained through the joint reinforcement of group norms. This allows for insights that would not otherwise be accessible to the subjects operating alone, as the inner parts and their interaction are in large part out of our own awareness. The group insight is then used to offer alternative and appropriate (and sometimes reparative and rewarding) models for interactions, for the "I" of each group member, and at the same time, for those inner parts operating between and within the sub-selves of the individual members.

Chris Farmer
March 2003

Bibliography

Schwartz, R.C. (1995) *Internal Family Systems Therapy.* New York: The Guildford Press

Chazan, R. (2001) *The Group as Therapist.* London: Jessica Kingsley